# ECG Assessment and Interpretaton

# ECG Assessment and Interpretation

## Bradford C. Lipman, MD

Assistant Clinical Professor
Department of Medicine
Medical College of Georgia
Augusta, Georgia

Clinical Cardiology
Cardiac Disease Specialists
Atlanta, Georgia

## Toni Cascio, RN, MN, CCRN

Clinical Educator
Adult Critical Care
Ochsner Foundation Hospital
New Orleans, Louisiana

F. A. DAVIS COMPANY • Philadelphia

F. A. Davis Company
1915 Arch Street
Philadelphia, PA 19103

Printed in Canada

Last digit indicates print number: 10 9 8 7 6 5 4 3 2

*Publisher, Nursing:* Robert G. Martone
*Production Editor:* Gail Shapiro
*Cover Design By:* Donald B. Freggens, Jr.

To my father, Bernard S. Lipman, MD, FACC, for his never-ending encouragement, devotion, and love. To my family, Leslie Joy, Larry, Bob, and Bill for their support. To my colleagues in cardiology, especially Thomas F. Deering, MD, FACC, for his undaunted enthusiasm and desire for teaching; and to C. Richard Conti, MD, FACC, Chief, Division of Cardiology, University of Florida, for his dedication and inspiration to teaching and education in the field of cardiology.

**Bradford C. Lipman**

To my husband Charlie, whose unwavering love and support sustained me. To Raja W. Dhurandhar, MD, whose wisdom and gift for teaching inspired me. To my colleagues in nursing and education, whose dedication to their profession is a source of unending admiration.

**Toni Cascio**

# Preface

Assessment and interpretation of the electrocardiogram is a skill that must be practiced by increasing numbers of health care professionals and clinical support personnel in today's high-tech environment. The expansion of ECG monitoring beyond the realm of the critical care unit has fueled the demand for competent practitioners who must learn to 'read' the ECG, whether it is a conventional 12-lead electrocardiogram, a rhythm strip, or a continuous tracing.

Learning the intricacies of the electrocardiogram can be both challenging and rewarding. Through our experiences in teaching electrocardiography, we have come to appreciate the learner's desire for an easily understood explanation of this complicated subject. Therefore, in this book we have attempted to create a simple, user-friendly resource by incorporating the most salient characteristics of common ECG rhythms and 12-lead tracings with practical clinical tips. An explanation of *why* selected characteristics apply is also presented. A variety of concepts related to cardiac disorders, including their effects on the electrocardiogram and antidysrhythmic drug therapy are also discussed. Whenever possible, examples and figures are used to illustrate each rhythm or concept. For maximum benefit, the reader is encouraged to correlate the ECG clues with each rhythm strip or 12-lead ECG example.

Unit I describes fundamental skills and concepts that are woven throughout the rest of the book. Units II and III focus on rhythm strip identification of common dysrhythmias and heart blocks; therapeutic options are also listed. Unit IV describes pacemaker concepts and functions, while Units V and VI focus primarily on myocardial infarction and a variety of miscellaneous conditions and their effects on the 12-lead ECG; a summary of key points is found at the end of these units. Tables of common cardiac drugs and dosages, as well as the most recent ACLS protocols, can be found in the Appendices.

Our book examines ECG assessment and interpretation on a basic level. For an in-depth analysis of complex rhythms and concepts in electrocardiography, the reader may consult additional references.

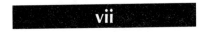

We hope that the reader finds this book a useful tool in the quest for competence in assessment and interpretation of the electrocardiogram.

**Bradford C. Lipman, MD, FACC**
**Toni Cascio, RN, MN, CCRN**

# Acknowledgments

The authors would like to express their deep appreciation to the following: To the patient staff of the F. A. Davis Company, particularly Bob Martone, Gail Shapiro, Herb Powell, and Ruth DeGeorge. To Patricia Gauntlett Beare, RN, PhD, for her encouragement and support. To our reviewers, whose comments and criticisms helped shape a better product. To our friends and colleagues in medical education, nursing, and clinical cardiology, without whose help this book would not have been possible.

For critical and timely review of the manuscript, we give special thanks to Bernard S. Lipman, MD, Professor Emeritus of Medicine (Cardiology), Emory University School of Medicine, and Thomas F. Deering, MD, electrophysiologist and colleague. We also wish to thank M. Daniel Byrd, MD, Linda Miller, RN, Brent Rodriguez, CCPT, and Edmund K. Kerut, MD, for their additional assistance. Also a special thank you from coauthor B.L. to coauthor T.C. for her hard work and energy in developing and producing this textbook.

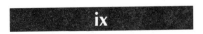

# Contents

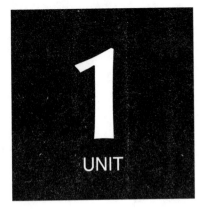

UNIT

# BASICS OF ECG INTERPRETATION

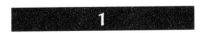

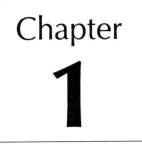

# Chapter 1

# INTRODUCTION TO THE ELECTROCARDIOGRAM

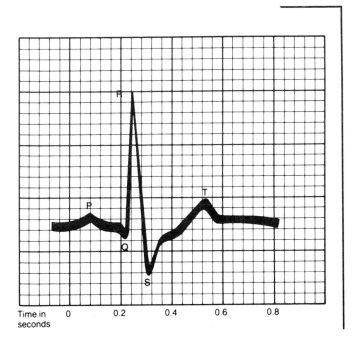

# HISTORY

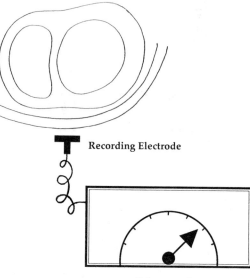

Recording Electrode

Galvanometer

**FIGURE 1–1.** Einthoven used a string galvanometer to record electrical currents from the human heart.

**ECG**

**galvanometer**

Welcome to the study of the electrocardiogram (ECG). The **ECG** is a graphic display of the electrical forces generated by the heart. Its history dates back to 1902, when Willem Einthoven recorded an electrical current from the human heart using an instrument called a string **galvanometer.** Since that time, electrocardiography has advanced in many different directions. Currently, the ECG is composed of 12 leads. It records the electrical impulses of the heart, as recorded from the surface of the body.

The ECG is commonly used to diagnose chamber enlargement, conduction abnormalities (heart block), dysrhythmias, myocardial infarction, drug effects, electrolyte alterations, and many other abnormalities. Further applications of more advanced ECG technology include exercise stress testing to diagnose coronary artery disease, Holter/telemetry monitoring and electrophysiologic testing to diagnose and treat dysrhythmias, signal-averaging of ECGs to help determine prognosis of dysrhythmias, and increasing uses of pacemaker technology.

**electro-cardiogram**

Welcome to the world of the **electrocardiogram.**

# ECG WAVEFORMS

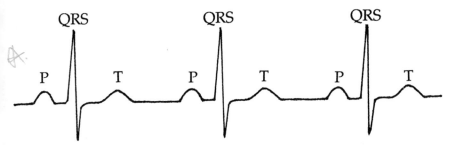

**FIGURE 1–2.** The P-QRS-T deflections recorded on ECG graph paper represent electrical activity in the atria and ventricles.

**waves**

**P-QRS-T**

The ECG records electrical impulses from the heart onto graph paper. These electrical impulses are recorded as **waves** or deflections that spread from the heart through the body to the surface electrodes.

Normally, one heartbeat is recorded as a grouping of waves called **P-QRS-T** deflections.

The P wave represents the electrical activity of the atria. When the atria are stimulated, the electrical impulses are recorded in the form of a P wave.

The QRS-T complex of waves represents the electrical activity of the ventricles. When the ventricles are stimulated, electrical impulses are recorded in the form of a QRS-T complex. This complex represents both electrical activation and electrical recovery of the ventricles.

# ACTIVATION OF THE ATRIA

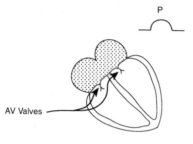

**AV Valves**

**FIGURE 1-3.** The P wave represents electrical activation (depolarization) of atrial muscle cells. The waveform that represents electrical recovery (repolarization) of atrial muscle cells is usually not visible on the ECG.

**P wave**

**depolarization**

When the atria are electrically activated, ECG electrodes record this activation as a deflection called the **P wave.** Electrical activation of heart muscle cells is caused by an electrical process called **depolarization.** When depolarization of atrial muscle cells occurs, a P wave is recorded on the ECG.

**repolarization**

After the atrial muscle cells have been depolarized (electrically activated), a reverse electrical process occurs to return the atrial muscle cells to their initial state. This reverse electrical process is called **repolarization.** Although atrial muscle cell repolarization is recorded as a deflection on the ECG, the waveform is usually buried or lost in the much larger QRS complex.

# ATRIAL PUMP

Depolarization = P wave      Mechanical contraction = atrial kick

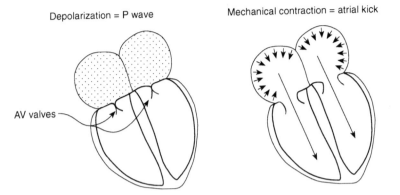

AV valves

**FIGURE 1–4.** Depolarization of atrial muscle cells, an electrical event, produces a P wave on the ECG (note that the AV valves are closed). Mechanical contraction of the atria follows immediately; blood is pumped past open AV valves into the ventricles (the atrial kick).

**depolarization**

**atrial kick**

**electrical
activation
contraction**

**Depolarization** of the atrial muscle cells results in activation of these cells. The atrial muscle cells contract together to pump blood into the ventricles. This event is called the **atrial kick**.

The ECG records depolarization of the atrial muscle cells by recording the **P wave**.

Remember, the P wave represents only **electrical activation**. **Contraction** of the atrial muscle cells and **pumping** of blood from the atria to the ventricles immediately follow atrial activation or depolarization.

The P wave represents an **electrical** event (depolarization of the atria). **Contraction** is the resultant mechanical event after activation (depolarization) has taken place.

# ACTIVATION OF THE VENTRICLES

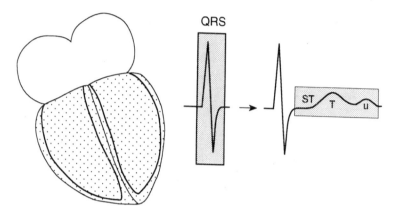

**FIGURE 1-5.** The QRS complex represents depolarization of ventricular muscle cells. The ST segment and T wave represent repolarization of these cells; the u wave may represent additional repolarization.

**QRS complex
depolarization**

When the ventricles are electrically activated, ECG electrodes record the activation as a deflection called the **QRS complex.** Electrical activation of ventricular muscle cells is caused by the process of **depolarization.** When depolarization of muscle cells in the ventricles occurs, a QRS complex is recorded on the ECG.

Immediately after depolarization of the ventricular muscle cells, the reverse electrical process occurs to return the ventricular muscle cells to their initial state. This reverse process is called **repolarization.** Repolarization of ventricular muscle cells is recorded on the ECG as the **ST segment** and accompanying **T wave.** Thus, repolarization of the ventricles is represented on the ECG as the **ST segment-T wave.**

**repolarization**

**ST segment
T wave**

Occasionally, a small deflection following the T wave may be seen. This is referred to as a u wave. It is believed to represent additional repolarization and may be found with hypokalemia (reduced body potassium). Its significance is unknown.

# THE VENTRICLES AS A PUMP

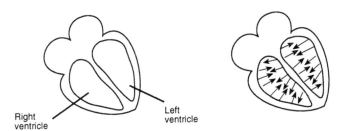

Depolarization = QRS Complex          Mechanical contraction = ventricular pumping

Right ventricle          Left ventricle

**FIGURE 1-6.** Depolarization of ventricular muscle cells produces a QRS complex on the ECG. Mechanical contraction of the ventricles follows immediately.

**Depolarization contract, pump**

**QRS complex**

**Depolarization** of the ventricular muscle cells results in activation of these cells. The ventricular muscle cells normally **contract** together to **pump** blood.

The ECG records depolarization of the ventricular muscle cells by recording the **QRS complex.**

Remember, the QRS complex represents electrical activation. **Contraction** of the ventricular muscle cells and **pumping** of blood from the ventricles to the lungs and to the rest of the body normally follows activation or depolarization.

The QRS complex represents an **electrical** event (depolarization of the ventricles). **Contraction** is the resultant mechanical event after activation (depolarization) has taken place.

# ANATOMY OF THE ATRIA

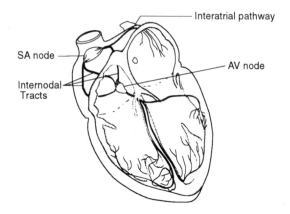

FIGURE 1-7. The heart's electrical impulse normally originates spontaneously from the SA node located high in the right atrium. It travels along special conduction pathways in the right and left atria. Atrial muscle cells are then activated in an organized fashion. (Adapted from Brown, KR and Jacobson, S: Mastering Dysrhythmias: A Problem-Solving Guide. FA Davis, Philadelphia, 1988, p 4, with permission.)

**SA node**

Normally, the heart's electrical impulse originates in the sinoatrial (SA) node. The **SA node** is located in the upper part of the right atrium. Electrical impulses originate spontaneously from the SA node to activate (depolarize) the muscle cells of the atria.

The electrical impulse from the SA node travels through three conducting pathways (anterior, middle, and posterior internodal pathways) in the right atrium to the atrioventricular (AV) node. An additional interatrial pathway called Bachmann's bundle transmits the electrical impulse to the left atrium. These pathways transmit the electrical impulse to the atrial muscle cells.

The atrial muscle cells are activated (depolarized) in an organized fashion as the impulse travels through these specialized atrial conducting pathways. Depolarization of atrial muscle cells produces the P wave on the ECG.

# AV NODE

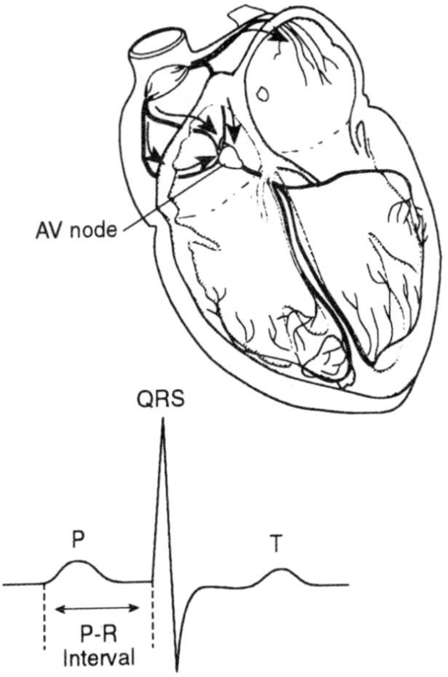

FIGURE 1-8. Impulses from the special atrial conduction pathways converge in the AV node (AV junction). The impulse is slowed in the AV node to allow time for the atria to contract and pump blood into the ventricles. AV delay is assessed by examining the PR interval on the ECG. (Adapted from Brown, KR and Jacobson, S: Mastering Dysrhythmias: A Problem-Solving Guide. FA Davis, Philadelphia, 1988, p 4, with permission.)

**AV node**

**PR interval**

The three internodal atrial conducting pathways meet at the atrioventricular node (**AV node,** AV junction). The AV node acts as a "way station" (delay area) in which impulses from the atria are slowed down. This delay of the impulse in the AV node allows time for the atria to contract and to pump blood into the ventricles.

The time interval from the beginning of the P wave to the beginning of the QRS complex is called the **PR interval.** It represents the time it takes for the atria to depolarize (P wave) and the normal delay of the impulse in the AV node. The PR interval also includes the short period of time for conduction into the ventricles up to the point of ventricular depolarization (QRS complex).

# ANATOMY OF THE VENTRICLES

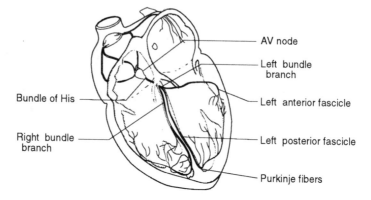

**FIGURE 1–9.** The electrical impulse emerging from the AV node travels through the Bundle of His, then down the bundle branches. The impulse travels into the right ventricle via the right bundle branch and into the left ventricle via the left bundle branch. Note that the left bundle branch divides into the left anterior fascicle and the left posterior fascicle. The impulse terminates in Purkinje fibers in the ventricles. Ventricular muscle cells are then activated in an organized fashion. (Adapted from Brown, KR and Jacobson, S: Mastering Dysrhythmias: A Problem-Solving Guide. FA Davis, Philadelphia, 1988, p 4, with permission.)

**bundle of His**

After the delay in the AV node, the impulse enters a short pathway called the **bundle of His.** The bundle of His splits into two important conducting pathways called the right bundle branch and the left bundle branch.

**right bundle branch**

**Purkinje fibers**

The **right bundle branch** conducts the impulse to the right ventricle. It divides into smaller branches and then into a special conducting network called the Purkinje system. **Purkinje fibers** conduct the impulse to the muscle cells in the right ventricle.

**left bundle branch fascicles**

The **left bundle branch** separates into two parts— the **anterior and posterior divisions** (fascicles)—that supply the left ventricle. The anterior fascicle transmits the impulse to the anterior portion of the left ventricle. The posterior fascicle transmits the impulse to the posterior portion of the left ventricle.

Both anterior and posterior fascicles conduct the impulse into the Purkinje system. Purkinje fibers conduct to the muscle cells in the left ventricle.

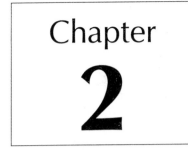

# Chapter 2

# ECG ELECTRODES AND LEADS

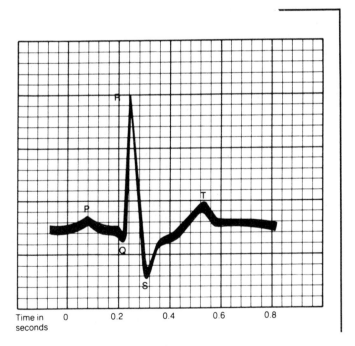

Time in seconds

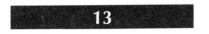

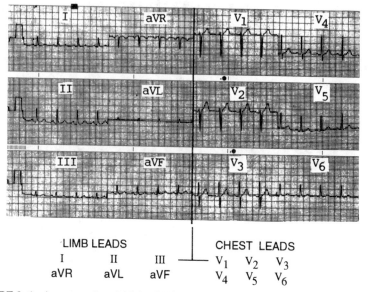

**FIGURE 2–1.** A conventional 12-lead ECG records electrical activity in the heart from 12 different views. There are six limb leads and six chest leads. (Adapted from Lipman, BC and Lipman, BS: ECG Pocket Guide. Year Book Medical Publishers, Chicago, 1987, p 7, with permission.)

**12-lead ECG**

The standard **12-lead ECG** is composed of 12 leads that record the electrical activity in the heart from 12 different views. Each ECG lead provides a unique picture of the electrical impulses transmitted from the heart to the surface of the body.

**limb leads**
**electrodes**

Of the 12 leads, six are designated as **limb leads.** They are derived from **electrodes** placed on or adjacent to the four limbs. The limb leads are designated I, II, III, aVR, aVL, and aVF.

**chest leads**

The other six leads are designated **chest** or **precordial leads** because they are derived from six electrodes placed on specific areas of the chest overlying the precordium (heart). The chest leads are designated $V_1$, $V_2$, $V_3$, $V_4$, $V_5$, and $V_6$.

# ELECTRODE PLACEMENT—LIMB ELECTRODES

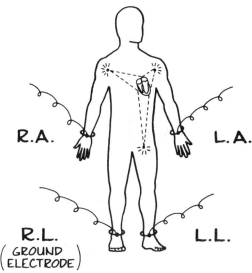

**FIGURE 2-2.** Limb electrodes are placed on the wrists and ankles, or, alternatively, on the shoulders and lower abdomen (at the junction of each limb with the body). (Adapted from Lipman, BC and Lipman, BS: ECG Pocket Guide. Year Book Medical Publishers, Chicago, 1987, p 8, with permission.)

**limb electrodes**

The recording **limb electrodes** are placed on the right arm (RA), left arm (LA), and left leg (LL). The right leg (RL) electrode is a ground (or neutral) electrode.

The limb electrodes actually record electrical forces from the heart as viewed from the **junction** of that limb with the body (i.e., at the shoulder and hip areas). The electrodes could be placed below each shoulder and above each groin to obtain the same tracings.

The **limb electrodes** have standard color-coded designations:

- Right arm (RA), white
- Left arm (LA), black
- Right leg (RL), green
- Left leg (LL), red

# ELECTRODE PLACEMENT—CHEST ELECTRODES

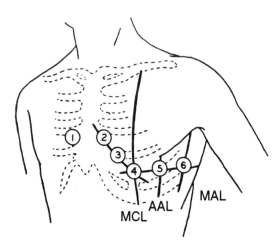

**FIGURE 2–3.** The six chest electrodes ($V_1$ through $V_6$) are placed on the anterior chest wall. (Adapted from Lipman, BC and Lipman, BS: ECG Pocket Guide. Year Book Medical Publishers, Chicago, 1987, p 8, with permission.) MCL = midclavicular line, AAL = anterior axillary line, MAL = midaxillary line

**chest**
**precordial**

The recording **chest** or **precordial** electrodes are placed on specific areas of the chest wall. Incorrect placement of the chest electrodes may turn what should have been a normal ECG tracing into an abnormal one. The standard six chest electrode sites are as follows:

$V_1$: Fourth intercostal space, right sternal border

$V_2$: Fourth intercostal space, left sternal border

$V_3$: Fifth intercostal space, midway between $V_2$ and $V_4$

$V_4$: Fifth intercostal space, midclavicular line

$V_5$: Fifth intercostal space, anterior axillary line

$V_6$: Fifth intercostal space, midaxillary line

# WHERE THE BIPOLAR LIMB LEADS COME FROM

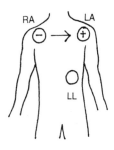 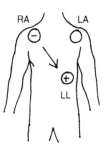 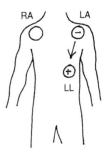

| Lead I | Lead II | Lead III |

FIGURE 2-4. Bipolar limb leads I, II, and III record electrical forces viewed between two electrodes, one designated positive and the other designated negative.

**limb electrodes**

**limb leads**

**bipolar leads**

Once the **limb electrodes** are placed on the body surface, the electrical forces from the heart are conveyed from the body to the ECG machine. The electrical forces are then displayed in six **limb leads** designated I, II, III, aVR, aVL, and aVF.

The first three leads (I, II, and III) are called **bipolar leads.** These leads use two electrodes at a time to record the tracing. For each bipolar lead, one limb electrode is arbitrarily **positive** (+) and the other arbitrarily **negative** (−). Bipolar leads record electrical forces generated from the two electrodes.

By convention, the two electrodes used to form each lead are:

**Lead I**

**Lead II**

**Lead III**

**Lead I:** Left arm positive (+) and right arm negative (−)

**Lead II:** Left leg positive (+) and right arm negative (−)

**Lead III:** Left leg positive (+) and left arm negative (−)

Remember, each bipolar limb lead records the electrical forces generated from the two designated electrodes.

# WHERE THE UNIPOLAR LIMB LEADS COME FROM

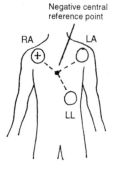
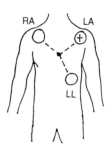
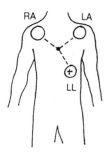

Lead aVR                    Lead aVL                    Lead aVF

**FIGURE 2-5.** Unipolar limb leads aVR, aVL, and aVF record electrical forces between a positive limb electrode and a negative central reference point created electronically.

**unipolar limb
leads
aVR, aVL, aVF**

The same **limb electrodes** are also used to form the three **unipolar limb leads.** They are designated by the letters "a" for augmented and "V" for unipolar, as leads **aVR, aVL, and aVF.** They are called unipolar because each lead uses only one electrode at a time to record the electrical forces generated from the heart. For each unipolar limb lead, the specific limb electrode is the positive (+) electrode, which records the electrical forces in relation to a negative central reference point created electronically. The "a" stands for augmented because the electrical forces recorded by the limb electrodes are electronically enlarged.

The unipolar limb electrodes used to form each unipolar limb lead are:

aVR: Right arm (RA) electrode (+)

aVL: Left arm (LA) electrode (+)

aVF: Left leg (LL) electrode (+)

Remember, the positive (+) electrode for each lead is that particular limb electrode (right arm positive in aVR, left arm positive in aVL, left leg positive in aVF).

# WHERE THE CHEST LEADS COME FROM

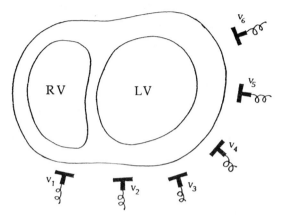

**FIGURE 2-6.** Unipolar chest leads V₁ through V₆ record electrical forces between a positive chest electrode and a negative central reference point created electronically.

**chest electrodes**
**chest leads**

The six **chest** (precordial) **electrodes** are used to record the six **chest leads.** The chest leads are unipolar, designated by the letter "V," as $V_1$, $V_2$, $V_3$, $V_4$, $V_5$, and $V_6$. Similar to the unipolar limb electrodes, each unipolar chest electrode is the **positive** (+) electrode, which records the heart's electrical forces in relation to a **negative** (−) central reference point.

It is important to place the chest electrodes in their proper positions for accurate recording of the chest leads (see p 16), especially when taking serial tracings.

# CONTINUOUS MONITORING

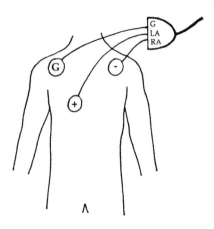

## Lead MCL$_1$

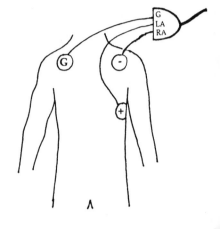

## Lead MCL$_6$

**FIGURE 2-7.** When using a 3-lead monitoring system, modified chest leads MCL$_1$ through MCL$_6$ are created by placing the positive electrode (LA) in the desired precordial position (see Fig. 2-3); the negative electrode (RA) is placed under the left clavicle, and the ground electrode (G) is placed under the right clavicle.

**continuous**

In the hospital setting, **continuous** bedside monitoring of the ECG is often performed. One or more leads may be monitored continuously from the bedside.

**three-electrode**

A **three-electrode** monitoring system uses one electrode designated as positive ($+$), one electrode designated as negative ($-$), and the third electrode as a ground. One limb lead at a time (I, II, or III) may be monitored by placing the positive and negative electrodes in their appropriate positions (see p 15) while keeping the ground electrode stationary, usually just underneath the right clavicle.

Using a three-electrode monitoring system, chest leads may be created for continuous monitoring by placing the positive electrode in the appropriate chest electrode location (see p 16) and by placing the negative electrode under the left clavicle. This is termed a **modified chest lead (MCL)**

**modified chest lead (MCL)**. Leads MCL$_1$ through MCL$_6$ may be obtained by placing the positive electrode in the appropriate chest electrode position.

**five-electrode**

A **five-electrode** monitoring system uses the four limb electrodes (RA, LA, RL, LL) in the conventional locations, with the fifth electrode being placed in the desired $V_1$ through $V_6$ position. Using this system, any one (or more) of the 12 leads may be continuously monitored from the bedside.

# UNCONVENTIONAL LEADS FOR EVALUATING ATRIAL ACTIVITY

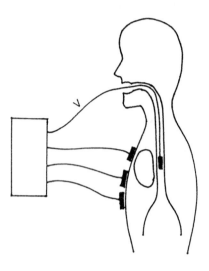

**FIGURE 2–8.** Unconventional leads like the esophageal lead depicted are used to magnify P waves. The V lead is attached to a special wire or nasogastric tube with an exploring electrode on the distal tip (the electrode may be imbedded in a gel cap). The tip is advanced into the esophagus until it rests behind the atria. Since the recording electrode is in close proximity to the atria, P waves appear larger than usual on the ECG.

**unconventional leads**

When analyzing rhythms, one should first search for the **P waves.** P waves (atrial activity) may occasionally be difficult to visualize on the ECG. If P waves (or any atrial activity, flutter waves, and so on) cannot be readily seen on the conventional 12-lead ECG, **unconventional leads** can be created for a more adequate assessment of atrial activity.

The unconventional leads include:

- Lewis lead: RA electrode placed in second intercostal space at right sternal border and LA electrode placed in fourth intercostal space at right sternal border; record from lead I
- Esophageal lead: Electrode wire (V lead) placed inside a nasogastric tube (or specially designed NG tube with an electrode embedded in a gelatin capsule on the tip); tip advanced into the esophagus approximately 25 to 30 cm in order to place it close to the atria; record from V lead to generate excellent display of atrial activity

- Intra-atrial lead: Specially designed electrode wire (V lead) advanced intravenously (usually from the internal jugular, subclavian, or femoral vein) into the right atrial cavity; record from inside the right atrium to generate excellent display of atrial activity

# Chapter

# 3

# GENERATION OF ECG WAVEFORMS

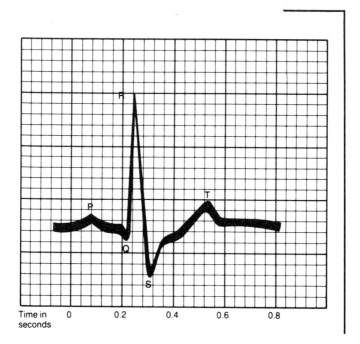

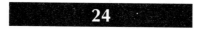

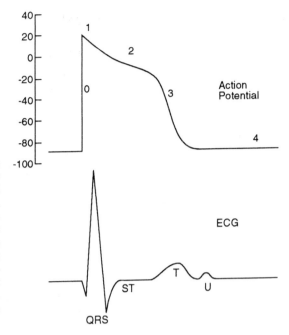

**FIGURE 3-1.** The action potential is an electrical process that precedes mechanical contraction of muscle cells. The phases of the action potential (0, 1, 2, 3, 4) correlate with waveforms recorded on the ECG. (Adapted from Beare, PG and Myers, JL: Principles and Practice of Adult Health Nursing. CV Mosby, St. Louis, 1990, p 765, with permission.)

**electrical event**

**action potential**

An electrical impulse precedes each heartbeat (mechanical contraction). The ECG records only the **electrical event** that is the stimulus for mechanical contraction.

Each muscle cell in the heart (and throughout the body) is stimulated to contract by going through an electrical process called the **action potential.** The action potential process is composed of five phases (0, 1, 2, 3, 4). The ECG records the summation of the action potentials of the muscle cells in the atria and ventricles as P-QRS-T waveforms.

It is important to understand the action potential process in order to understand how normal ECG waveforms are generated. Knowledge of this process also helps to explain how drugs (especially antidysrhythmic drugs), electrolyte disorders (e.g., high or low potassium levels), and other conditions may alter components of the ECG.

# ACTION POTENTIAL OF A MUSCLE CELL AT REST, PHASE 4

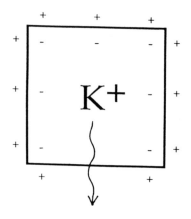

Na+

Ca++

**FIGURE 3-2.** In a resting (or polarized) muscle cell, the cations sodium (Na) and calcium (Ca), located primarily on the outside of the cell, are unable to cross the cell wall. The cation potassium (K), located primarily on the inside of the cell, leaks slowly across the cell wall to the outside. The charge on the outside of the cell is positive. The charge on the inside of the cell is negative. The resting state of a muscle cell correlates with phase 4 of the action potential.

**charged**
**polarized**
**action potential**

**Cations**

**sodium**
**calcium**

**phase 4**

Normally at rest, each muscle cell is **charged** or **polarized.** The outside of the muscle cell is positively charged and the inside is negatively charged. The **action potential** is directly related to the difference between the outside and inside charges.

**Cations** are positively ($+$) charged particles (ions) that help to generate the action potential. At rest, outside the cell, the cations **sodium** (Na) and **calcium** (Ca) predominate. These cations are unable to cross into the cell at rest. Inside the cell, the cation potassium (K) predominates. At rest, potassium leaks slowly to the outside of the cell. This slow loss of positive potassium ions from the inside to the outside of the cell causes the interior of the cell to be negative ($-$) relative to the outside of the cell, which is positive ($+$).

The movement of ions while the muscle cell is at rest is called **phase 4** of the action potential. During phase 4, potassium slowly leaks to the outside of the cell, causing the inside of the cell to be negative ($-$) relative to the outside of the cell, which is positive ($+$).

# DEPOLARIZATION, PHASE 0 OF THE ACTION POTENTIAL

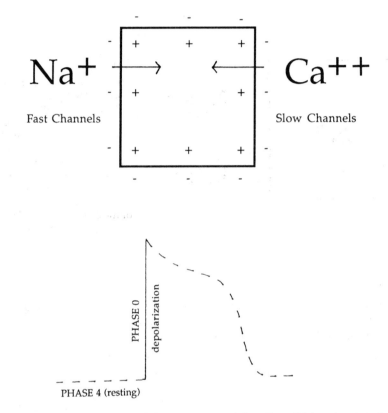

**FIGURE 3–3.** During phase 0 of the action potential, sodium (Na) rushes into the cell through pathways called fast channels, and calcium (Ca) enters the cell through pathways called slow channels. The charge on the inside of the cell changes from negative to positive, and depolarization begins. The waveforms recorded on the ECG represent depolarization of muscle cells.

**phase 0**

**fast channels**
**slow channels**

When a muscle cell at rest is stimulated (activated), the inside of the cell suddenly becomes positive ($+$) and the outside negative ($-$). This change, **phase 0** of the action potential, is caused by the rapid inward rush of sodium cations from the outside to the inside of the cell. Sodium enters the cell through pathways or gates called **fast channels.** During phase 0 of the action potential, another set of pathways or gates called **slow channels** opens to allow calcium cations to slowly enter the cell.

depolarization

P wave

QRS complex

The influx of both sodium and calcium into the cell causes the inside of the cell to become positive (+) relative to the outside (−).

The rapid change of polarity on the inside and outside of the cell during phase 0 is called **depolarization**. During depolarization, the muscle cell is activated to contract. *Depolarization is the electrical process that is recorded on the ECG.*

In the muscle cells of the atria, phase 0 of the action potential (depolarization) correlates with the **P wave** on the ECG. In the muscle cells of the ventricles, phase 0 of the action potential (depolarization) correlates with the **QRS complex** on the ECG.

# REPOLARIZATION, PHASES 1, 2, AND 3 OF THE ACTION POTENTIAL

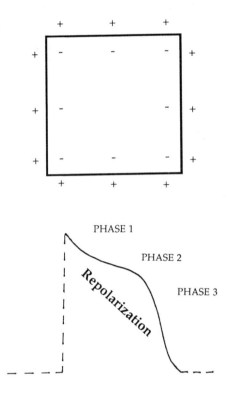

**FIGURE 3-4.** Phases 1, 2, and 3 of the action potential represent repolarization, or recovery, of the cells. The inside of the cell changes from positive back to its original resting negative charge.

**repolarization**

Immediately after **depolarization** (phase 0 of the action potential), the muscle cell returns to its previous resting state through a process called **repolarization.** The process of repolarization is also recorded on the ECG.

Phases 1, 2, and 3 of the action potential form the repolarization phenomenon. The polarity of the muscle cell is restored so that the outside of the cell is again positively charged and the inside negatively charged.

The three phases of repolarization are:

Phase 1: The fast sodium channels suddenly close, but the slow calcium channels remain open.

**ST segment**

Phase 2 (plateau phase): The continued flow of calcium into the cell is balanced by the flow of potassium to the outside of the cell. Phase 2 correlates with the **ST segment** on the ECG.

**T wave**

Phase 3: The calcium channels close, but potassium continues to leak to the outside. Phase 3 correlates with the **T wave** on the ECG.

When the repolarization process has been completed, the cell is ready to be activated or depolarized again.

# PACEMAKER CELL ACTION POTENTIAL

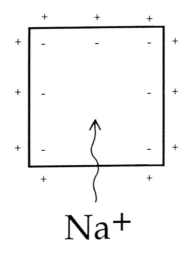

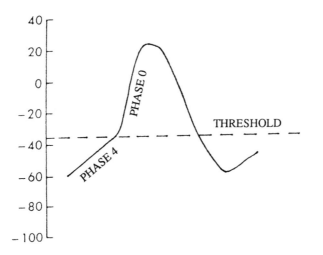

**FIGURE 3–5.** Pacemaker cells, unlike muscle cells, do not require a stimulus to depolarize; in other words, they are capable of spontaneous depolarization. During resting phase 4, potassium (K) leaks to the outside the cell, and sodium (Na) leaks to the inside of the cell. When a critical voltage threshold is reached, depolarization (phase 0) begins as calcium (Ca) enters the cell through slow channels. (Bottom portion adapted from Beare, PG and Myers, JL: Principles and Practice of Adult Health Nursing. CV Mosby, St. Louis, 1990, p 766, with permission.)

**Pacemaker cells**

**Pacemaker cells,** located primarily in the SA node but also in other areas of the heart, initiate the electrical impulses that activate the muscle cells. Pacemaker cells are called **automatic** cells because they initiate impulses **spontaneously.** The processes of depolarization and repolarization (action potential) are different in pacemaker cells as compared with muscle cells.

In the resting pacemaker cell, phase 4 of the action potential (resting phase) still involves a slow leak of potassium from the inside to the outside of the cell. However, sodium from outside the cell gradually leaks into the cell at the same time, a phenomenon that does not occur in the muscle cell.

**threshold**

As sodium leaks into the cell during phase 4, a critical voltage **threshold** is reached. When this critical threshold is reached, phase 0 of the action potential (depolarization) begins spontaneously.

Depolarization (phase 0) of the pacemaker cell is caused by influx of calcium into the cell through slow channels. Sodium entry by fast channels does *not* occur in pacemaker cells as it does in muscle cells.

The repolarization process (phases 1, 2, and 3) in pacemaker cells is similar to muscle cells so that spontaneous depolarization may occur again.

# CLINICAL IMPORTANCE OF THE ACTION POTENTIAL

| Antidysrhythmic Agents Classified by Mechanism of Action | |
| --- | --- |
| Class I | Block Na channels |
| Class II | Beta blockers |
| Class III | Block multiple phases of the action potenial |
| Class IV | Calcium channel blockers |

**FIGURE 3-6.** The four classes of antidysrhythmic agents and their mechanisms of action.

**slow cells**

**fast cells**

**action potential**

**ectopic**

Pacemaker cells are described as **slow cells** because their depolarization is dependent on calcium entry into the cells through **slow channels.** Muscle cells are described as **fast cells** because their depolarization is dependent on sodium entry into the cells through **fast channels.**

Many drugs used to treat dysrhythmias alter certain phases of the **action potential.** Their specific mechanism of action may slow or retard the usual processes of depolarization and repolarization to prevent or treat dysrhythmias.

Specific calcium channel blocking agents (class IV antidysrhythmic agents; see p 250) inhibit the slow channels in pacemaker cells. This results in a *decrease in heart rate* in patients taking these agents.

The class I antidysrhythmic agents (see p 250) inhibit the fast sodium channels in muscle cells. This effect inhibits phase 0 depolarization of the muscle cells to suppress **ectopic** impulses.

Class III antidysrhythmic agents (see p 250) alter several phases of the action potential, and their exact mechanism of action is not known at this time.

# RECORDING DEPOLARIZATION AS A WAVE

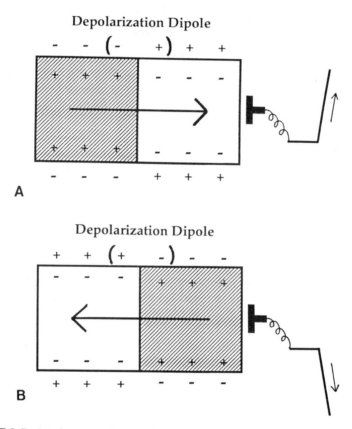

**FIGURE 3-7.** An electrode placed adjacent to a muscle cell records depolarization as either a positive or a negative deflection, depending on the location of the electrode in relation to the depolarization dipole. A depolarization dipole is a moving pair of charges, with the positive charge leading the way. (*A*) When the depolarization dipole moves toward a recording electrode, a positive deflection is recorded on the ECG. (*B*) When the depolarization dipole moves away from a recording electrode, a negative deflection is recorded on the ECG.

**dipole**

**depolarization dipole**

During depolarization of a muscle cell, the outside positive charge changes to negative (see action potential, p 27). As the electrical stimulus travels through the cell, a moving pair of charges called a **dipole** is created. This dipole consists of a positive (+) charge followed by a negative (−) charge. This **depolarization dipole** has the positive (+) charge leading the activation wave.

When an electrode is placed adjacent to the cell, the depolarization dipole can be recorded as a waveform or deflection. By convention, an **upright deflection** represents positive (+) movement toward the electrode. A **downward deflection** represents movement away from the electrode. The upward or downward deflection of a wave depends on which part of the dipole is facing the electrode and its direction of movement.

When the depolarization dipole is moving toward the electrode, a positive, or upward, deflection is recorded. In this situation, the positive head of the dipole is moving toward the electrode.

When the depolarization dipole travels away from the electrode, a negative, or downward, deflection is recorded. In this situation, the electrode "sees" the negative end, or tail, of the dipole moving away from it.

# RECORDING REPOLARIZATION AS A WAVE

### Repolarization Dipole

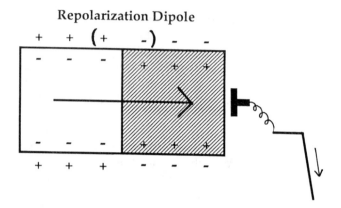

**FIGURE 3–8.** An electrode placed adjacent to a muscle cell records repolarization as either a positive or a negative deflection, depending on the location of the electrode in relation to the repolarization dipole. A repolarization dipole is a moving pair of charges, with a negative charge leading the way (opposite from the depolarization dipole). In this example, the repolarization dipole is moving toward a recording electrode, so the deflection on the ECG is negative (the electrode sees the negative head of the dipole moving toward it).

**repolarization dipole**

During repolarization ("recharging") of the muscle cell, the outside negative charge changes back to positive. As this electrical process travels through the cell, an opposite pair of charges, called a **repolarization dipole,** is created. This dipole (opposite of depolarization dipole) consists of a negative (−) charge followed by a positive (+) charge. It has a negative (−) charge leading the wave of repolarization.

When the repolarization dipole moves toward the electrode, a negative, or downward, deflection is recorded. This is because the negative (−) head of the dipole is moving toward the electrode.

When the repolarization dipole travels away from the electrode, a positive, or upward, deflection is recorded as the negative tail of the dipole is moving away.

BOX 3-1 **Recording Depolarization and Repolarization**

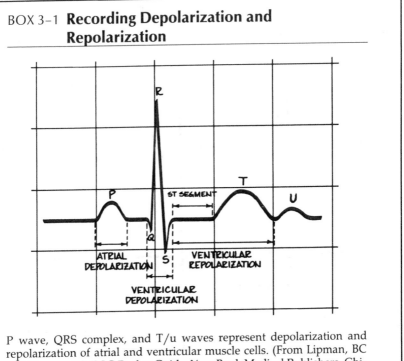

P wave, QRS complex, and T/u waves represent depolarization and repolarization of atrial and ventricular muscle cells. (From Lipman, BC and Lipman, BS: ECG Pocket Guide. Year Book Medical Publishers, Chicago, 1987, p 21, with permission.)

# P WAVE

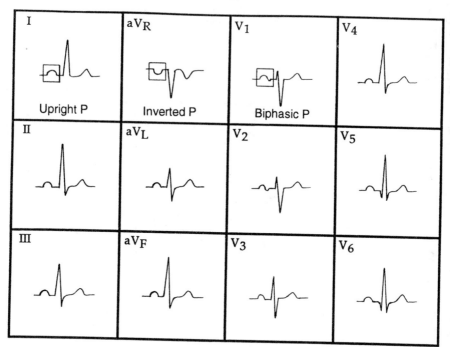

**FIGURE 3–9.** P waves appear upright (positive), inverted (negative), or biphasic, depending on the lead.

**P wave**

The **P wave** represents depolarization of atrial muscle cells. Its contour results from sequential activation of the right atrium (where the SA node is located), then the left atrium. A P wave normally precedes each QRS complex. The waveform representing repolarization of the atria is usually not seen on the ECG because it is small and usually buried within the much larger QRS complex.

**P wave characteristics.** The P wave is normally positive (above the baseline) in leads I, II, aVF, and $V_4$ through $V_6$. It is usually negative (below the baseline) in lead aVR. The P wave is **biphasic** (part of the P wave is above the baseline and part is below) in leads III,

**biphasic**

aVL, and $V_1$ through $V_3$. A normal P wave is gently rounded, not peaked or notched. Its height is normally less than 3 mm, and its width is normally less than 0.11 second.

# QRS COMPLEX

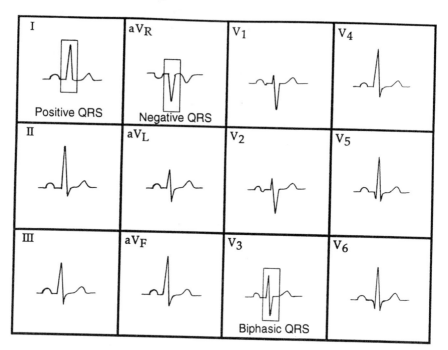

**FIGURE 3-10.** The QRS complex appears upright (positive), inverted (negative), or biphasic, depending on the lead.

**QRS complex**

The **QRS complex** represents depolarization of ventricular muscle cells. Its contour results from the nearly simultaneous depolarization of both the right and left ventricles. The QRS complex normally follows each P wave.

**QRS complex characteristics.** The normal QRS complex is predominantly positive (above the baseline) in leads that "look" at the heart from the left side (I, aVL, $V_5$, $V_6$) and in leads that look at the inferior or underside of the heart (II, III, aVF). It is negative (below the baseline) in leads that look at the heart from the right side (aVR, $V_1$, $V_2$). The

QRS complex is biphasic (part above and part below the baseline) in leads $V_3$, $V_4$, and sometimes III.

The normal QRS complex is less than 25 mm high and less than 0.10 seconds in duration.

# QRS TERMINOLOGY

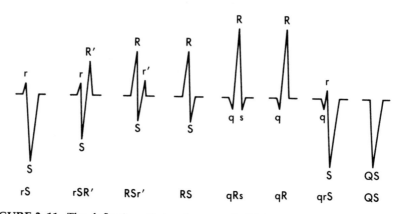

**FIGURE 3-11.** The deflections that make up each QRS complex can be labeled, as in the examples shown here (refer to text). (From Beare, PG and Myers, JL: Principles and Practice of Adult Health Nursing. CV Mosby, St. Louis, 1990, p 770, with permission.)

Each lead records depolarization of the ventricles as a QRS complex. The QRS complex can be composed of multiple deflections above and below the baseline, which are labeled. The large deflections are labeled with upper case (capital) letters and the small deflections with lower case (small) letters.

**Q wave.** First downward (or negative) deflection *preceding* an R wave

**R wave.** First upward (or positive) deflection

**S wave.** The downward or negative deflection that *follows* an R wave

**R' wave.** Second positive deflection

**S' wave.** Second negative deflection

# ST SEGMENT

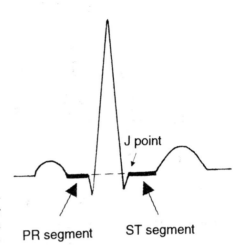

J point

PR segment     ST segment

**FIGURE 3-12.** The ST segment is normally isoelectric (deflected neither above nor below the baseline) when compared to the preceding PR segment.

**ST segment**

The **ST segment** represents the interval of time between the end of the QRS complex (a juncture called the J-point) and the beginning of the T wave. Though not a true waveform, the ST segment represents the beginning of ventricular repolarization. The shape and position relative to the baseline may be altered with episodes of ischemia, metabolic abnormalities, drug effects, and other conditions.

**isoelectric**

**ST segment characteristics.** The ST segment is normally **isoelectric** (neither above nor below the baseline compared with the preceding PR segment). Slight displacement of the ST segment above or below the baseline may represent a normal variant. Greater degrees of ST segment displacement may indicate ischemia, injury, strain, drug or metabolic effects, stroke, and many other conditions.

# T WAVE, u WAVE

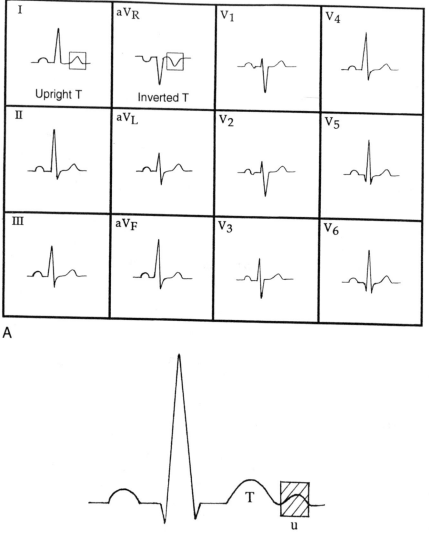

A

B

**FIGURE 3–13.** (*A*) The T wave is normally oriented in the same direction as the QRS complex. (*B*) The u wave may follow the T wave and is normally oriented in the same direction.

**T wave**

The **T wave** represents the end of repolarization of the ventricles and always follows the QRS complex (repolarization always follows depolarization).

**u wave**

The **u wave** is a small deflection following the T wave. Its significance is unknown, but it may represent further repolarization of the ventricles.

**T wave characteristics.** The T wave is normally oriented in the same direction as the QRS complex. It is slightly rounded and asymmetrical and usually exhibits a smooth takeoff from the end of the ST segment. Its configuration may be distorted by clinical conditions such as myocardial ischemia, hypertrophy, and metabolic abnormalities.

**u wave characteristics.** The u wave is usually observed in the chest leads. It may be upright in patients with hypokalemia or inverted in patients with ischemia or left ventricular hypertrophy.

---

BOX 3-2 **Intervals**

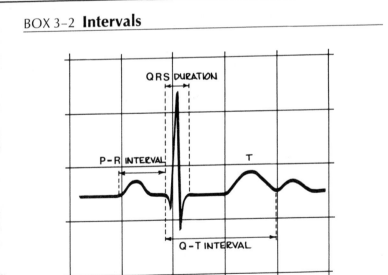

The PR interval, QRS interval, and QT interval represent the times required for depolarization and repolarization of muscle cells. (From Lipman, BC and Lipman, BS: ECG Pocket Guide. Year Book Medical Publishers, Chicago, 1987, p 24, with permission.)

# PR INTERVAL

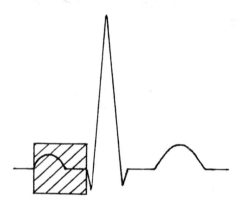

**FIGURE 3–14.** The PR interval is measured from the beginning of the P wave to the beginning of the QRS complex. The PR segment (measured from the end of the P wave to the beginning of the QRS complex) is not routinely measured; it is used as a baseline to assess ST segment displacement.

**PR interval**

The **PR interval** is measured from the beginning of the P wave to the beginning of the QRS complex. It represents the total amount of time required for depolarization of the atria (P wave) as well as the time required for the impulse to travel slowly through the AV junction, through the bundle branches, and just up to the point of ventricular depolarization (QRS complex).

**PR interval characteristics.** The normal PR interval ranges from 0.12 second to an upper limit of 0.20 second in the adult. Its duration shortens when the heart rate increases and lengthens when the heart rate decreases.

The PR interval may be shorter than normal (less than 0.12 second) in infants, in patients with an accessory or additional conduction pathway that bypasses the AV junction (see p 233), or in those taking certain drugs (eg, steroids)

The PR interval may be longer than normal (greater than 0.20 second) if conduction or depolarization is prolonged in the atria because of drug effect, hypertrophy, or atrial dilatation. The PR interval may also lengthen if conduction is slowed in the AV junction because of drug effect (digitalis, beta blockers, calcium channel blockers), degeneration with aging (sick sinus syndrome; see p 150), and myocardial infarction (especially inferior).

**PR Segment**

**Note:** The **PR segment** is the distance from the end of the P wave to the beginning of the QRS complex. It is used as a baseline to evaluate elevation or depression of the ST segment.

# QRS INTERVAL

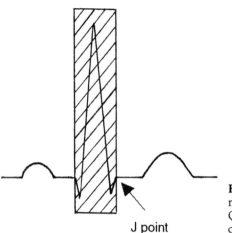

J point

FIGURE 3-15. The QRS interval is measured from the beginning of the QRS complex to the end of the QRS complex, at the J joint.

**QRS interval**
**J-point**

The **QRS interval** is measured from the beginning of the QRS complex to its end point, called the **J-point** (see p 43). The QRS interval represents the time required for depolarization of both ventricles.

**QRS interval characteristics.** The normal QRS interval is less than 0.10 second in any lead. It may be slightly wider in the chest leads ($V_1$ through $V_6$) than in the limb leads because the chest leads record the brief time required for depolarization of the septum, which is often not visible in the limb leads.

The QRS interval may widen to greater than 0.10 second when there is delayed conduction through the bundle branches or fascicles (see Chapter 12), abnormal or aberrant conduction within the ventricles such as with ventricular premature complexes (VPCs; see p 120), or early and abnormal activation of the ventricles through an accessory or bypass tract (see p 233).

A short QRS interval (less than 0.08 second) is normal.

# QT INTERVAL

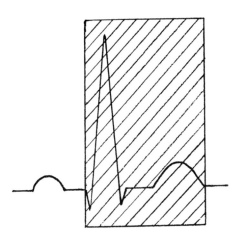

**FIGURE 3-16.** The QT interval is measured from the beginning of the QRS complex to the end of the T wave.

QT interval

The **QT interval** represents the total time required for both **depolarization and repolarization** of the ventricles to occur. It is measured from the beginning of the QRS complex to the end of the T wave.

**QT interval characteristics.** The normal QT interval ranges from 0.35 to 0.45 second. The length of the QT interval normally varies according to age, gender, and especially heart rate. As the heart rate increases, the QT interval decreases; conversely, as the heart rate decreases, the QT interval increases. The normal QT interval, corrected for heart rate, is found in Box 3–3.

If the QT interval is prolonged, serious dysrhythmias such as torsade de pointes (p 137) may arise. Electrolyte abnormalities and certain antidysrhythmic drugs can prolong the QT interval.

## BOX 3–3 QT Interval: Upper Limits of Normal

| Heart Rate per Minute | Men and Children (Sec) | Women (Sec) |
|---|---|---|
| 40 | 0.49 | 0.50 |
| 45 | 0.47 | 0.48 |
| 50 | 0.45 | 0.46 |
| 55 | 0.43 | 0.44 |
| 60 | 0.42 | 0.43 |
| 65 | 0.40 | 0.42 |
| 70 | 0.39 | 0.41 |
| 75 | 0.38 | 0.39 |
| 80 | 0.37 | 0.38 |
| 85 | 0.36 | 0.37 |
| 90 | 0.35 | 0.36 |
| 95 | 0.35 | 0.36 |
| 100 | 0.34 | 0.35 |

From Lipman, BC and Lipman, BS: ECG Pocket Guide, Year Book Medical Publishers, Chicago, 1987, with permission.

# BASICS OF R WAVE PROGRESSION

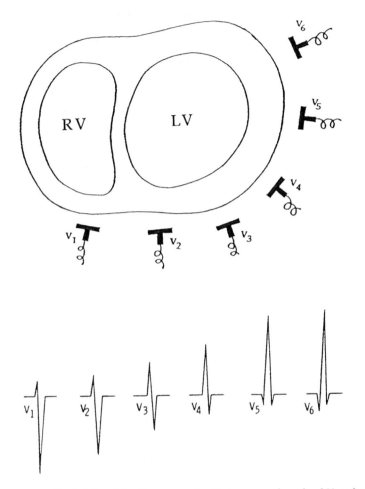

**FIGURE 3-17.** The height of the R wave gradually increases from lead $V_1$ to lead $V_6$, a phenomenon called R wave progression. [RV = right ventricle; LV = left ventricle.] (*Bottom* from Chung, EK: Electrocardiography: Practical Applications with Vectorial Principles, ed. 3. 1985, Appleton & Lange, Norwalk, CT, p 33, with permission.)

R wave progression is the gradual increase in height of the R wave (of the QRS complex) as chest leads $V_1$ to $V_6$ are recorded on the ECG. Abnormal R wave progression (from chest leads $V_1$ to $V_6$) may indicate myocardial infarction, obstructive lung disease, hypertrophy (thickening) or dilatation of the ventricles, or other cardiac disease states. The six chest electrodes must be placed in their correct positions (see p 16). *Incorrect placement of the electrodes may turn what should have been a normal ECG tracing into an abnormal one.*

The left ventricle normally has two to three times the mass of the right ventricle. Thus depolarization of the left ventricle contributes to the majority of the QRS deflection. Also, the left ventricle lies *to the left and behind* the right ventricle. Notice the placement of the six chest electrodes in relation to the ventricles. The right-sided electrodes are $V_1$ and $V_2$. The left-sided electrodes are $V_5$ and $V_6$. Normally, depolarization of the ventricles (represented by the QRS complex) is recorded as an increasingly positive, upright deflection (taller R wave) as leads $V_1$ to $V_6$ are recorded.

# SPECIFICS OF R WAVE PROGRESSION

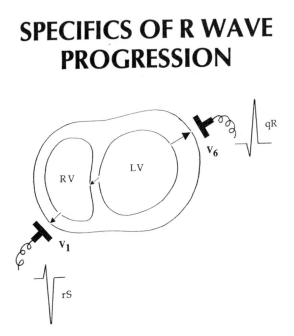

**FIGURE 3-18.** The initial portion of the QRS complex represents depolarization of the septum. The remainder of the QRS complex represents depolarization of the right and left ventricles. Since the left ventricle is much larger than the right, most of the QRS complex reflects depolarization forces recorded from the larger left ventricle. In lead $V_1$, septal depolarization is represented by a small r wave; the rest of the QRS is negative because depolarization forces are moving away from the recording electrode. In lead $V_6$, septal depolarization is represented by a small q wave; the rest of the QRS is positive because depolarization forces are moving toward the recording electrode. [RV = right ventricle; LV = left ventricle.]

To understand more about R wave progression, remember how electrical impulses are conducted through the ventricles. After the electrical impulse emerges from the AV junction, it travels through the bundle of His and then down the right and left bundle branches. Normally the left side of the ventricular septum is depolarized first. Depolarization of the septum is directed from the left to the right side.

The impulse then travels quickly through the bundle branches and fascicles (see p 12) to Purkinje fibers. Depolarization of the right and left ventricular free walls then occurs.

The initial portion of the QRS deflection (in chest leads $V_1$ to $V_6$) represents depolarization of the septum. The balance of the QRS complex represents depolarization of the ventricular free walls, the majority of which is contributed by the left ventricle.

The right-sided chest leads ($V_1$, $V_2$) look at the heart from the right side. They see depolarization of the septum (activation from the left side to the right side) as current flowing toward them. The initial part of the QRS complex in leads $V_1$ and $V_2$ is recorded as a small positive wave, the septal r wave. The remainder of depolarization in the ventricles is produced by activation of the left ventricle as current flows away from electrodes $V_1$ and $V_2$. Thus, the remainder of the QRS complex is negative, creating a large S wave as current is seen moving away from these electrodes.

Leads $V_5$ and $V_6$ are left-sided chest leads that look at the ventricles from the left side. They see depolarization of the septum (normally left side to right side) as current flowing away from them. The initial part of the QRS complex in these leads is recorded as a small negative deflection, the septal q wave. The remainder of ventricular depolarization is contributed by the larger left ventricle. Thus, these left-sided electrodes record this large amount of current directed toward them as a large positive deflection, the R wave.

# ABNORMAL R WAVE PROGRESSION

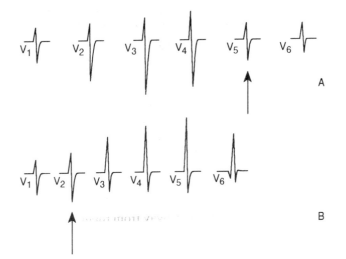

**FIGURE 3–19.** When R wave progression is normal, transition from a predominantly negative to a predominantly positive QRS complex occurs at lead $V_3$ or $V_4$ (see Fig. 3–17). Abnormal R wave progression means that this transition occurs in other leads. (*A*) In poor R wave progression, transition occurs later than expected, in leads $V_5$ or $V_6$ (arrow), and/or the R waves fail to increase in size in leads $V_1$, $V_2$, and $V_3$. (*B*) In early transition, the QRS becomes predominantly positive in leads $V_1$ or $V_2$ (arrow).

The normal gradual increase in R wave height as leads $V_1$ to $V_6$ are examined is called R wave progression. The transition from a predominantly negative ($\dashv\!\!\!\backslash$) QRS complex to a predominantly positive ($\dashv\!\!\!\perp$) QRS complex usually occurs in leads $V_3$ or $V_4$ (see Fig. 3–17).

**Poor R wave progression (PRWP)**

**Poor R wave progression (PRWP)** occurs if the QRS complex does not become predominantly positive by lead $V_4$ or if the R waves in $V_1$ through $V_3$ remain small and do not progressively increase in size. PRWP may be seen with anterior or septal myocardial infarction, left ventricular hypertrophy, and other disease states.

**Early transition**

**Early transition** occurs when the QRS complex becomes predominantly positive earlier than normal, in leads $V_1$ or $V_2$. This may be found with posterior myocardial infarction, right ventricular hypertrophy, or as a normal variant in infants.

R wave progression may also appear to be abnormal if the chest electrodes are placed incorrectly.

# Chapter

# 4

# PACEMAKERS AND HEART RATES

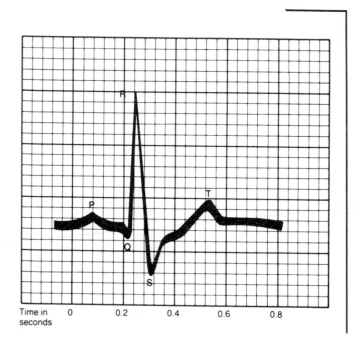

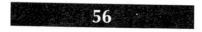

**automaticity**

The heart's dominant pacemaker is the sinoatrial (SA) node. Located high in the right atrium, the SA node independently initiates the driving electrical impulse. This ability to initiate impulses spontaneously is called **automaticity** (see p 32).

Other potential pacemaker sites located in the heart also have the property of automaticity. These sites are located in the atria, atrioventricular (AV) junction, and ventricles and are usually dormant. However, they contain **automatic** pacemaker cells, which can initiate impulses independently, usually at slower rates than the SA node. These other pacemaker sites are normally usurped by the faster SA node (sinus) pacemaker.

# NORMAL PACEMAKER RATES

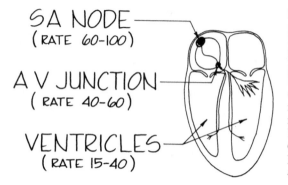

SA NODE
( RATE 60-100 )

A V JUNCTION
( RATE 40-60 )

VENTRICLES
( RATE 15-40 )

FIGURE 4-1. The dominant pacemaker is in the SA node. Escape pacemakers in the AV junction and ventricles fire at progressively slower rates. Under normal conditions, the escape pacemakers are overridden by the faster sinus pacemaker. (From Lipman, BC and Lipman, BS: ECG Pocket Guide. Year Book Medical Publishers, Chicago, 1987, p 46, with permission.)

Normally, automatic pacemaker cells in the SA node generate impulses at a rate of between 60 and 100 beats per minute (bpm). If the SA node fails to generate an impulse, then a lower **escape** pacemaker site (in the AV junction or ventricles) takes over. These lower escape pacemaker sites act like electrical backups that fire at slower rates.

**escape**

The lower escape pacemaker sites have a slower intrinsic rate of discharge. The **AV junction** has an intrinsic rate of **40 to 60 bpm**. If the AV junction takes over at the rate of 40 to 60 bpm when the SA node has failed, it is called **junctional escape rhythm.**

**AV junction**
**40 to 60 bpm**

**Ventricular pacemaker cells**
**15 to 40 bpm**

**Ventricular pacemaker cells** have an intrinsic rate of discharge of **15 to 40 bpm**. If impulses above the ventricles (supraventricular impulses) fail to reach the ventricles, the ventricles may fire at a rate of 15 to 40 bpm. This is called a **ventricular escape rhythm.**

# ECG GRAPH PAPER

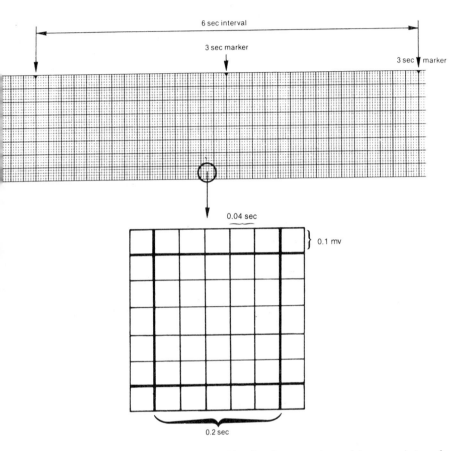

**FIGURE 4–2.** ECG graph paper. The width of each square is used to assess intervals of time; large squares equal 0.2 second, and small squares equal 0.04 second. The height of each square is used to assess voltage; large squares equal 0.5 mv (or 5 mm), and small squares equal 0.1 mv (or 1 mm). (Adapted from Brown, KR and Jacobson, S: Mastering Dysrhythmias: A Problem-Solving Guide. FA Davis, Philadelphia, 1988, p 9, with permission.)

| | |
|---|---|
| **ECG graph paper** | **ECG graph paper** is composed of horizontal and vertical lines with light lines and dark lines that intersect to form small and large squares, respectively. Horizontal measurements reflect units of time; vertical measurements reflect measurements of voltage. Each **small** |
| **small square** | **square** equals 1 mm, 0.04 second in width, 0.1 millivolt |

**large square**        (mV) in height. Each **large square** equals 5 mm, 0.20
second in width, 0.5 mV in height.

The **standard speed** for recording the ECG is 25
mm/sec. A faster recording speed (50 mm/sec) is occasionally used to visualize wave deflections better.

# ECG STANDARDIZATION

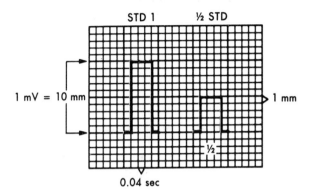

**FIGURE 4-3.** Standardization is adjusted to increase or decrease the size of the QRS in order to make ECG interpretation easier. At STD 1 (the normal standardization), a box 1 mV in height is recorded (equals 2 large squares or 10 mm). At 1/2 STD, a box 0.5 mV in height is recorded (equals 1 large square or 5 mm). At STD 2 (not shown), a box 2 mV in height is recorded (equals 4 large squares or 20 mm). (Adapted from Beare, PG and Myers, JL: Principles and Practice of Adult Health Nursing. CV Mosby, St. Louis, 1990, p 769, with permission.)

**standardized**    The ECG is **standardized** for accurate measurement of voltage in the vertical direction. A special signal is inscribed into the recording. The standard signal is a 1-mV deflection 10 mm high. With this standard, 1 mm in height equals 0.1 mV. This is known as Std 1.

Occasionally, when there is severe hypertrophy or thickening of the ventricles, the voltage or height of the QRS deflection is extremely high with the normal standardization. Adjusting the standard to one half (Std ½) will decrease the height so that 5 mm equals 1.0 mV. By doubling the standard to Std 2, 20 mm equals 1.0 mV, which may allow easier interpretation of previously smaller waveforms.

# CALCULATION OF HEART RATE: 1500 METHOD

**1500 method**

Heart rate is calculated as the number of heartbeats per minute. Heart rate usually implies ventricular rate (the number of QRS complexes per minute), but it can also refer to atrial rate (the number of P waves per minute). In both cases, three methods may be used to calculate heart rate. For teaching purposes, ventricular rate will be calculated.

**The 1500 method,** the most precise way to determine heart rate, can be used only if the rhythm is regular (no irregular beats seen).

**How To:**   Count the number of small squares between two consecutive QRS complexes. Because there are 1500 small squares per minute (0.04 second per square), divide the number of small squares into 1500. This result equals heart rate per minute.

**Hint:**   To save time, create a chart that can be used for at-a-glance calculation of heart rate (see box 4-1).

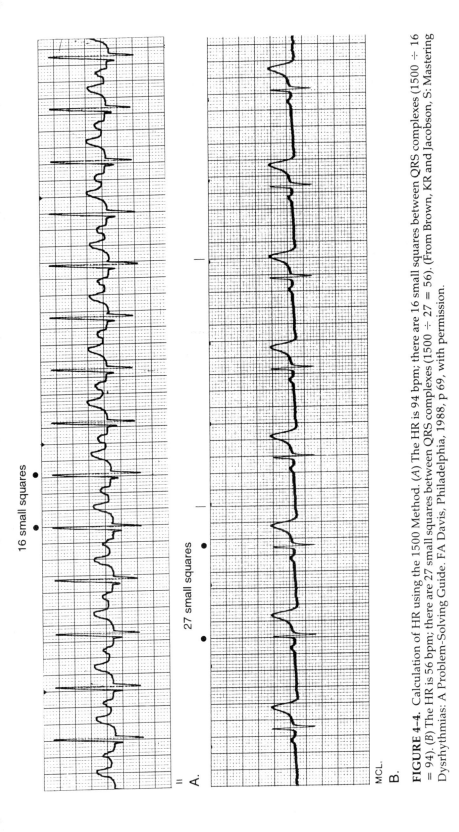

**FIGURE 4-4.** Calculation of HR using the 1500 Method. (*A*) The HR is 94 bpm; there are 16 small squares between QRS complexes (1500 ÷ 16 = 94). (*B*) The HR is 56 bpm; there are 27 small squares between QRS complexes (1500 ÷ 27 = 56). (From Brown, KR and Jacobson, S: Mastering Dysrhythmias: A Problem-Solving Guide. FA Davis, Philadelphia, 1988, p 69, with permission.

BOX 4–1 **Calculation of Heart Rate: 1500 Method and R-R Method**

| Number of Small Squares Between R Waves | Heart Rate |
|:---:|:---:|
| 5 | 300 |
| 6 | 250 |
| 7 | 214 |
| 8 | 188 |
| 9 | 167 |
| 10 | 150 |
| 11 | 136 |
| 12 | 125 |
| 13 | 115 |
| 14 | 107 |
| 15 | 100 |
| 16 | 94 |
| 17 | 88 |
| 18 | 83 |
| 19 | 79 |
| 20 | 75 |
| 21 | 71 |
| 22 | 68 |
| 23 | 65 |
| 24 | 62 |
| 25 | 60 |
| 26 | 58 |
| 27 | 56 |
| 28 | 54 |
| 29 | 52 |
| 30 | 50 |
| 31 | 48 |
| 32 | 47 |
| 33 | 45 |
| 34 | 44 |
| 35 | 43 |
| 36 | 42 |
| 37 | 41 |
| 38 | 39 |
| 39 | 38 |
| 40 | 37 |

# CALCULATION OF HEART RATE: R-R METHOD

**R-R method**

The **R-R method** is quick and easy, but for it to be accurate the heart rhythm must be regular. It is a variation of the 1500 method and requires minimal calculation.

**How To:** Find a QRS where the peak of the R wave falls on a heavy dark line. Use this QRS as a reference. If the next QRS falls on the very next dark line, the rate is 300 bpm. The distance between the two QRS complexes is five small boxes. The heart rate is 1500 divided by 5 equals 300 bpm. If the distance between two QRS complexes is two heavy lines (10 small boxes), the heart rate is 1500 divided by 10 equals 150 bpm. If the interpreter can remember the heart rate at each heavy line (between two consecutive QRS complexes), the heart rate can be calculated rapidly. Those important heart rate numbers are 300, 150, 100, 75, 60, and 50.

**Hint:** Remember the numbers 300, 150, 100, 75, 60, and 50, corresponding to each heavy line, for a quick calculation of heart rate.

**Another Hint:** If the two consecutive QRS complexes do not fall evenly on two heavy lines, use a piece of paper to mark off the two complexes. Then, place the first mark on a heavy black line and count down, as before, to the next mark. If the second mark is between heavy lines, then an average or estimate between the two corresponding heart rate numbers may be calculated.

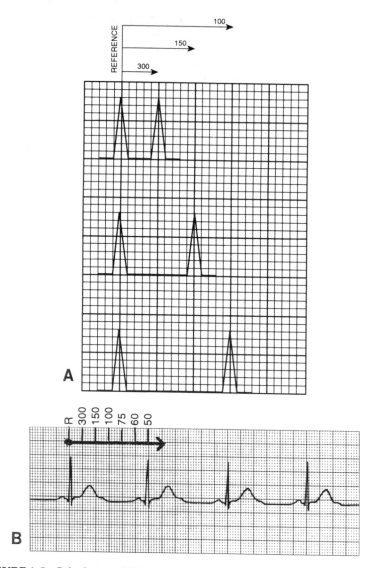

**FIGURE 4–5.** Calculation of HR using the R-R Method. (*A*) Any QRS whose peak falls on a dark line can be used as a reference. If the next QRS falls on the next dark line, the HR is 300 (or, 1500 ÷ 5 = 300). If it falls on the second dark line, the HR is 150 (or, 1500 ÷ 10 = 150). If it falls on the third dark line, the HR is 100 (or, 1500 ÷ 15 = 100). (*B*) In this example, the HR is 50 bpm. The first QRS complex on the strip falls on a dark line and is used as a reference. The next QRS falls on the sixth dark line to the right, corresponding to a rate of 50 (or, 1500 ÷ 30 = 50). (*B* From Wilson, RF: Critical Care Manual: Applied Physiology and Principles of Therapy, ed 2. FA Davis, Philadelphia, 1992, p 130, with permission.)

# CALCULATION OF HEART RATE: 6-SECOND METHOD

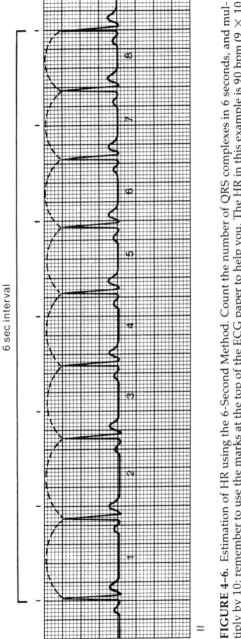

**FIGURE 4–6.** Estimation of HR using the 6-Second Method. Count the number of QRS complexes in 6 seconds, and multiply by 10; remember to use the marks at the top of the ECG paper to help you. The HR in this example is 90 bpm (9 × 10 = 90). (From Brown, KR and Jacobson, S: Mastering Dysrhythmias: A Problem-Solving Guide. FA Davis, 1988, p 9, with permission.)

**6-second
method**

The **6-second method** is the easiest but least accurate approach for calculating heart rate. It provides an estimate and is useful when the rhythm is irregular.

**How To:**  Note the short vertical lines or dots at the top of the ECG graph paper. These usually represent 1-, 2-, or 3-second intervals. Simply count the number of QRS complexes occurring in 6 seconds and multiply the result by 10 (6 seconds times 10 equals 60 seconds). That product equals the heart rate per minute.

# Chapter

5

# QRS AXIS

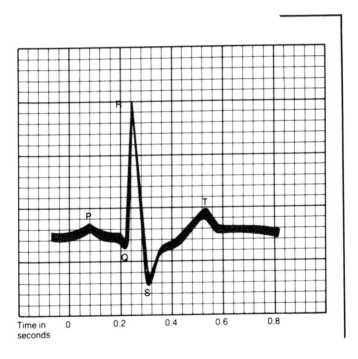

Time in
seconds

0        0.2       0.4      0.6      0.8

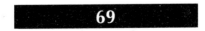

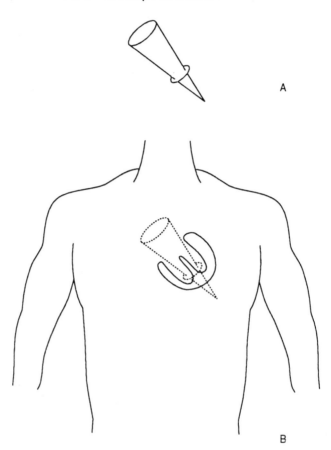

**FIGURE 5–1.** (*A*) Axis can be depicted as an arrow with both length and direction. (*B*) The QRS axis represents the main direction of current flow during depolarization of the ventricles. The normal QRS axis in an adult points downward and toward the left.

**QRS axis**

**Axis** represents the direction of electrical forces in the heart. An **arrow** that has both length and direction can be used to depict axis. It is important to determine the main direction of current flow during depolarization of the ventricles **(QRS axis)** in every 12-lead ECG. An abnormal QRS axis may occur with hypertrophy of the ventricles, myocardial infarction, conduction block in the ventricles, and multiple other causes.

The P wave axis, ST axis, and T wave axis may also be determined, but this is not done routinely. The QRS axis, however, should be calculated in *every* 12-lead ECG.

# LEAD AXIS

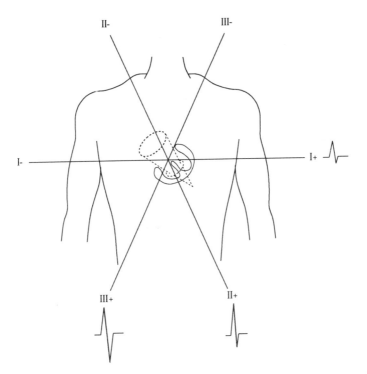

**FIGURE 5-2.** The shape of the QRS complex is different in each lead because each lead looks at depolarization in the ventricles from a different perspective. Note how the QRS complex looks different in each of the three leads illustrated.

The **QRS axis** represents the major direction of depolarization in the ventricles. It is determined by analyzing the shape of the QRS complex in each lead. The deflections of the QRS complex may be predominantly positive (above the baseline), predominantly negative (below the baseline), biphasic (equal amount above and below the baseline), or very small in size.

The shape of the QRS complex in each specific lead depends on the direction of depolarization in the ventricles as recorded in that lead. Each lead records a QRS complex with a particular shape because each lead "looks at" the heart from a different direction. The direction of ventricular depolarization in each lead is

**lead axis**

called **lead axis.** The total QRS axis is determined by examining each of the lead axes.

Note that each lead is oriented in a certain direction in relation to the heart (see p 74). Also, each lead has a positive (+) and a negative (−) end.

# HEXAXIAL REFERENCE SYSTEM

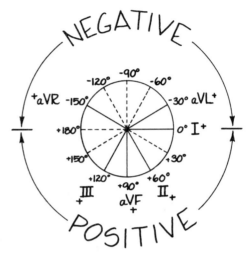

**FIGURE 5-3.** The hexaxial reference system, also called the axis wheel, intersects the lead axes of the six limb leads at a common center point. Note that the positive and negative ends of each lead axis are assigned specific degrees on the wheel (negative in the upper half, positive in the lower half). (From Lipman, BC and Lipman, BS: ECG Pocket Guide. Year Book Medical Publishers, Chicago, 1987, p 38, with permission.)

**hexaxial**
**reference**
**system**

The **hexaxial reference system** neatly places all six limb leads together into one picture so that **QRS axis** may be determined.

The end points of each lead axis in this "axis wheel" are assigned degrees ranging from 0° to 180°, positive in the lower half of the wheel and negative in the upper half.

Each lead axis in this system has a negative and a positive end. It is helpful to memorize the location of each lead's positive end on the axis wheel.

The positive ends of lead axes I, II, and III are located at 0°, +60°, and +120°, respectively.

The positive ends of lead axes aVR, aVL, and aVF are located at −150°, −30°, and +90°, respectively.

# LOCALIZING LEADS

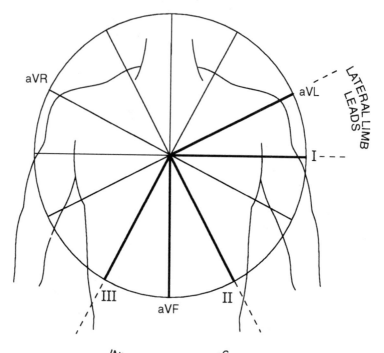

**FIGURE 5-4.** In the hexaxial reference system, limb leads I and aVL are directed laterally (lateral limb leads); limb leads II, III, and aVF are directed inferiorly (inferior limb leads).

**lateral limb leads**

**inferior limb leads**

Imagine placing the hexaxial reference system with all six lead axes directly on top of the body. The positive ends of leads I (0°) and aVL (−30°) are directed toward the left or lateral side of the heart. These leads are termed **lateral limb leads.**

The positive ends of leads II (+60°), III (+120°), and aVF (+90°) are directed toward the bottom or inferior side of the heart. These leads are termed **inferior limb leads.**

The positive end of lead aVR is directed toward the right side of the body.

# QRS AXIS: NORMAL AND ABNORMAL

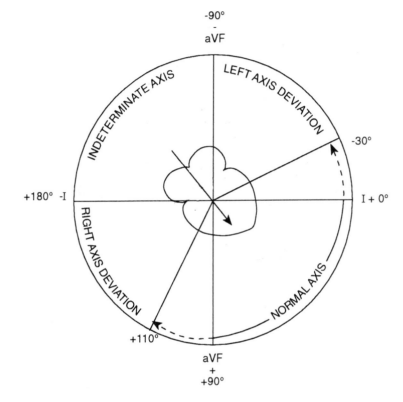

**FIGURE 5-5.** The axis wheel can be divided into four quadrants. A QRS axis that falls within a given quadrant can be labeled normal axis, left axis deviation, right axis deviation, or indeterminate axis. Note that a normal QRS axis may extend slightly beyond its quadrant boundaries.

**normal QRS axis**

**axis deviation**

The QRS axis represents the average direction of depolarization in the ventricles. The normal QRS axis in the adult points downward and to the left. On the hexaxial reference system, the **normal QRS axis** ranges between 0° and +90°, although normal can vary from −30° to +110°.

Abnormal QRS axis, called **axis deviation,** represents an abnormal direction of ventricular depolarization. Axis deviation may occur with myocardial infarction, congenital heart disease, ventricular hypertrophy or enlargement, fascicular block, and many other conditions.

Consider the axis wheel as a four-quadrant pie. The normal QRS axis points toward the left lower quadrant. If the QRS axis points to the left upper quadrant, it is termed **left axis deviation.** If the QRS axis points toward the right lower quadrant, it is termed **right axis deviation.** If the QRS axis points toward the right upper quadrant, it is termed extreme right axis deviation, indeterminant axis, or "no man's land."

**left axis deviation**

**right axis deviation**

# EVALUATION OF QRS AXIS IN LEAD I

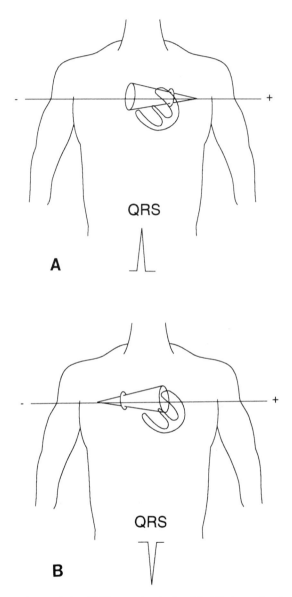

**FIGURE 5-6.** Analysis of the QRS complex in lead I. (A) A predominantly positive QRS complex results in a lead axis pointing toward the positive end of lead I. (B) A predominantly negative QRS complex results in a lead axis pointing toward the negative end of lead I.

(Continued on next page)

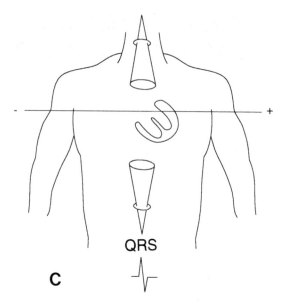

C

QRS

**FIGURE 5-6.** (*Continued*) (C) A small or biphasic QRS complex results in a lead axis pointing perpendicular to lead I.

**positive QRS**

**negative QRS**
**biphasic QRS**

If the main direction of depolarization in the ventricles (QRS axis) is toward the positive end of lead I, the QRS deflection in lead I will be predominantly **positive.** If the direction of depolarization is toward the negative end of lead I, the QRS deflection will be predominantly **negative.** If the direction is perpendicular to lead I, the deflection will be very small or **biphasic** (part above and part below the baseline).

The QRS deflection (positive *or* negative) is greatest when current flow is **parallel** to the lead axis. When current flow is **perpendicular** to the lead axis, the deflection is small or biphasic or both.

**FIGURE 5-7.** Estimation of the QRS axis using the Quadrant Method. (*A*) Examine lead I. The QRS in this example is positive, so the direction of current flow is toward the positive end of lead I; shade the two quadrants closest the positive end of lead I. (*B*) Examine lead aVF. The QRS in this example is positive, so the direction of current flow is toward the positive end of lead aVF; shade the two quadrants closest to the positive end of lead aVF. (*C*) The QRS axis falls in the quadrant where the two shaded quadrants overlap. In this example, the QRS axis is normal.

# DETERMINATION OF QRS AXIS: QUADRANT METHOD

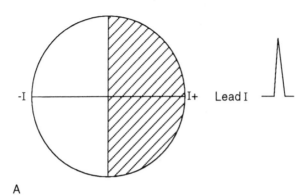

-I ——————— I+    Lead I

A

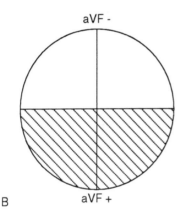

aVF -

Lead ᴀVF

B    aVF +

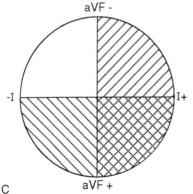

aVF -

-I ——————— I+    QRS axis is normal

C    aVF +

**quadrant method**

The **quadrant method** is the easiest and quickest way to determine QRS axis. It does not give a precise measurement but places the axis inside one of the four quadrants in the axis wheel. Estimation of axis using this method takes only seconds.

The only leads that need to be examined are leads I and aVF:

1. **Examine lead I.** If the QRS complex is predominantly positive, the direction of current flow is toward the positive end of lead I (or somewhere within the left upper or left lower quadrants). If the QRS is predominantly negative, the direction of current flow is toward the negative end of lead I (or somewhere within the right upper or right lower quadrants).

2. Shade the two quadrants corresponding to the direction of current flow in lead I.

3. **Examine lead aVF.** Apply the same method described for lead I and shade the two quadrants corresponding to the direction of current flow in lead aVF. If the QRS complex in lead aVF is predominantly positive, shade the two lower quadrants; if predominantly negative, shade the two upper quadrants.

4. The final estimate of QRS axis is located in the single shaded quadrant that overlaps.

# BOX 5-1 Normal Axis and Axis Deviation with the QRS Axis Estimated Using the Quadrant Method

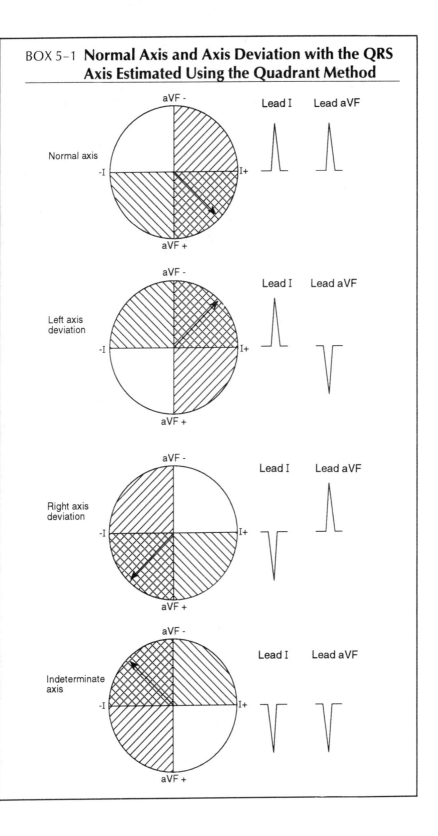

# DETERMINATION OF QRS AXIS: PERPENDICULAR METHOD

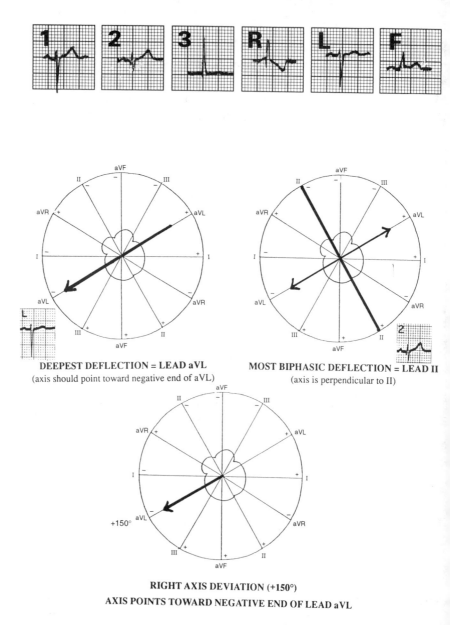

**DEEPEST DEFLECTION = LEAD aVL**
(axis should point toward negative end of aVL)

**MOST BIPHASIC DEFLECTION = LEAD II**
(axis is perpendicular to II)

**RIGHT AXIS DEVIATION (+150°)**
**AXIS POINTS TOWARD NEGATIVE END OF LEAD aVL**

**perpendicular method**

The **perpendicular method** is the most accurate method for determining QRS axis. It requires examining all six limb leads. The QRS axis is oriented toward the positive end of the lead axis that has the tallest positive deflection or toward the negative end of the lead axis that has the deepest negative deflection. Additionally, the axis points perpendicular to the lead axis with the smallest or most biphasic deflection.

1. Examine the QRS complex in all six limb leads. Look for the lead with the tallest positive deflection or the deepest negative deflection. If the QRS is predominantly positive, the axis points toward the positive end of that lead axis. If the QRS is predominantly negative, the axis points toward the negative end of that lead axis.
2. Next, look for the lead with the smallest or most biphasic (equally positive and negative) QRS deflection. The axis is oriented **perpendicular** to this lead. Perpendicular means at a 90° angle on either side of this lead axis. The initial lead used in point 1 shows which perpendicular side the QRS points toward, the positive side or the negative side.
3. To **fine tune** the QRS axis, look closely at the lead with the smallest or most biphasic deflection. If the QRS is slightly more positive than negative, the axis should be shifted slightly off the perpendicular toward the positive end of the lead axis. If the QRS is slightly more negative than positive, the axis should be shifted off the perpendicular toward the negative end of the lead axis.

←────────────────

**FIGURE 5–8.** QRS axis calculated using the Perpendicular Method. The lead with the largest deflection is lead aVL (deepest negative) so the axis should point toward the negative end of lead aVL. The lead with the smallest or most biphasic deflection is lead II (most biphasic); the axis points perpendicular to lead II and toward the negative end of lead aVL. The final QRS axis is +150°, or right axis deviation.

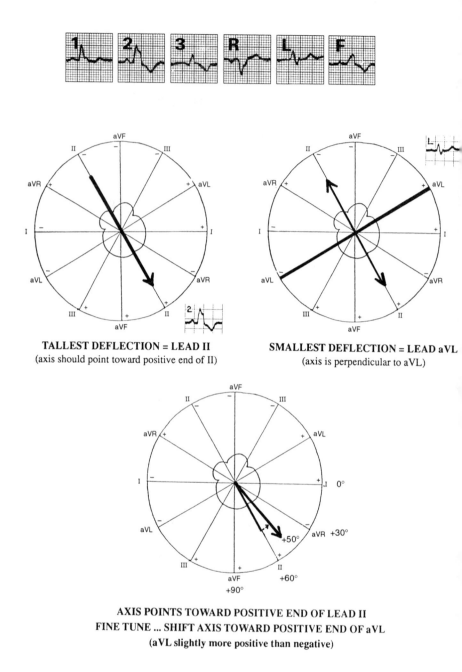

**TALLEST DEFLECTION = LEAD II**
(axis should point toward positive end of II)

**SMALLEST DEFLECTION = LEAD aVL**
(axis is perpendicular to aVL)

**AXIS POINTS TOWARD POSITIVE END OF LEAD II**
**FINE TUNE ... SHIFT AXIS TOWARD POSITIVE END OF aVL**
(aVL slightly more positive than negative)

**AXIS IS NORMAL (+50°)**

**FIGURE 5–9.** Normal axis calculated using the Perpendicular Method. The lead with the largest deflection is lead II (tallest positive) so the axis points toward the positive end of lead II. The lead with the smallest or most biphasic deflection is lead aVL (most biphasic); the axis points perpendicular to lead aVL, or toward the positive end of lead II. Since lead aVL is slightly more positive than negative, fine tune the QRS axis by shifting the axis slightly toward the postive end of lead aVL. The final QRS axis is +50°, normal axis.

# QRS AXIS DEVIATION

There are multiple causes for a change in the average direction of depolarization in the ventricles, which is called **QRS axis deviation.** Some causes of QRS axis deviation may be pathologic (e.g., acute myocardial infarction), whereas other causes may be more benign (e.g., aging), representing a normal variant. It is helpful to determine whether QRS axis deviation is sudden (accompanied by signs and symptoms of acute pathology) or has developed gradually over time. Comparison of present and past ECGs is usually helpful.

**Left axis deviation (LAD)** occurs when the QRS axis lies between −30° and −90°. Causes of LAD include left ventricular enlargement, left ventricular hypertrophy, aging process (normal variant with increasing age), myocardial infarction, left anterior fascicular block, and endocardial pacing.

**Right axis deviation (RAD)** occurs when the QRS axis lies between +90° and +180°. Causes of RAD include conditions that increase right ventricular work such as pulmonary hypertension, pulmonic stenosis, and acute pulmonary embolism. Other causes include right ventricular hypertrophy, congenital heart disease (atrial septal defect, tetralogy of Fallot, and so on), myocardial infarction, left posterior fascicular block, and epicardial pacing.

**Indeterminate axis** occurs when the QRS axis lies between +180° and −90°. This term is also used when the exact axis cannot be determined such as when all of the six limb leads are biphasic.

**Left axis deviation (LAD)**

**Right axis deviation (RAD)**

**indeterminate axis**

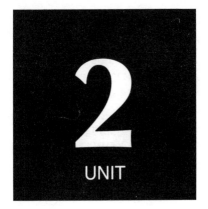

**2**

UNIT

# DYSRHYTHMIAS

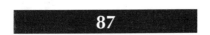

A **dysrhythmia** (also known as an **arrhythmia**) is an abnormal rhythm. It is any rhythm other than normal sinus rhythm. When assessing dysrhythmias, P waves and QRS complexes must be analyzed with respect to five basic parameters:

1. **Atrial rate (the P wave rate) and ventricular rate (the QRS rate).** Both atrial and ventricular rates should be identical.
2. **Regularity of P waves and QRS complexes.** P-P intervals (the distance between two consecutive P waves) and R-R intervals (the distance between two consecutive R waves) should be identical.
3. **Intervals.** The PR interval and QRS interval should be within normal limits.
4. **Relationship of P waves to QRS complexes.** There should be one P wave for every QRS complex.
5. **Presence of ectopic activity.** No premature or escape complexes should be noted.

Because determining the relationship between the P wave and the QRS complex is a critical step in rhythm interpretation, the astute clinician looks for the leads in which P waves are easily visible. P waves are usually seen best in the inferior leads (II, III, and aVF) and in chest leads $V_1$ and $V_2$. QRS complexes are readily visible in all leads. Moreover, the **morphology** (shape) of P and QRS waveforms may provide clues that enable the clinician to fine-tune the diagnosis. *It is often helpful to examine more than one lead before reaching a conclusion.*

It is essential to remember that the ECG reflects only *electrical* activity in the heart. To determine the *mechanical* consequences of dysrhythmias, clinical parameters such as the pulse and blood pressure must be assessed. Although it may be a simple matter to identify a dysrhythmia, do not stop there. *Always* remember to "treat the patient, not the ECG."

## ☐ PACEMAKER SITES AND HEART RATES

The sinoatrial (SA) node, located high in the right atrium, is the pacemaker site where cardiac impulses are normally initiated. If the SA node fails, then a lower **escape** pacemaker site in the atrioventricular (AV) junction or ventricles may take over to drive the heart.

Normally pacemaker cells in the SA node initiate electrical impulses that override other potential pacemakers in the heart. This is because the SA node normally possesses the fastest intrinsic rate of discharge. The lower escape pacemaker sites are usually depolarized by the faster sinus impulses. In adults, the normal sinus rate is 60 to 100 beats per minute (bpm). The next potential pacemaker site, the AV junction, initiates impulses at an intrinsic rate of 40 to

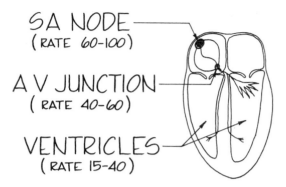

**FIGURE II-1.** Pacemaker sites and their inherent rates. The SA node is the dominant pacemaker, with an intrinsic rate between 60 and 100 per minute. The escape rate in the AV junction is between 40 and 60 per minute; the escape rate in the ventricles is between 15 and 40 per minute. (From Lipman, BC and Lipman, BS: ECG Pocket Guide. Year Book Medical Publishers, Chicago, 1987, p 46, with permission.)

60 bpm. If the SA node fails to discharge or if a sinus impulse fails to conduct, a junctional escape rhythm at 40 to 60 bpm normally takes over. Last, ventricular pacemaker cells possess an intrinsic rate of 15 to 40 bpm. If the higher supraventricular pacemaker sites fail to discharge or if those impulses cannot be conducted, a ventricular escape rhythm would normally take over at 15 to 40 bpm.

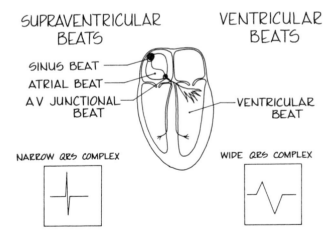

**FIGURE II-2.** Supraventricular versus ventricular origin. Rhythms originating above the ventricles are called "supraventricular," and those originating within the ventricles are called "ventricular." Normally supraventricular rhythms result in narrow QRS complexes, whereas those of ventricular origin result in wide QRS complexes. (From Lipman, BC and Lipman, BS: ECG Pocket Guide. Year Book Medical Publishers, Chicago, 1987, p 47, with permission.)

**CLINICAL TIP**

*Supraventricular dysrhythmias are rhythm disturbances that origi-
nate **above the ventricles,** in the SA node, the atria, or the AV junction (AV node).* Conduction within the ventricles usually remains
undisturbed, resulting in a narrow QRS complex.

**CLINICAL TIP**

*Ventricular dysrhythmias are rhythm disturbances that originate
**within the ventricles.*** Intraventricular conduction is abnormal,
resulting in a wide QRS complex.

# Chapter 6

# NORMAL SINUS RHYTHM
# AND VARIANTS

## ☐ NORMAL SINUS RHYTHM

In normal sinus rhythm (NSR), pacemaker impulses are initiated in the sinoatrial (SA) node, travel through the atrial pathways, and are delayed at the atrioventricular (AV) node. Depolarization of the atria produces a P wave. Impulse conduction proceeds unimpeded through the AV node and down the bundle branches to Purkinje fibers in the ventricles, causing ventricular depolarization and normally producing a narrow QRS complex.

### CHARACTERISTICS

1. The P wave is usually upright in leads II, III, aVF, and $V_1$. Its morphology remains constant at all times.
2. P-P and R-R intervals are equal and regular.
3. Atrial and ventricular rates are identical and range between 60 and 100 bpm.
4. There is no ectopic activity.

Sometimes during sinus rhythm, the morphology of the P waves or QRS complexes will appear abnormal. The PR and QRS intervals may also exceed normal limits. In such cases, the label "sinus rhythm" still applies, but one would hesitate to describe a rhythm as "normal" when abnormalities of waveform or interval exist.

### ☐ CLINICAL TIP
When it comes to ECG interpretation, it helps to be a creature of habit. Do not leave anything to chance, and *never assume anything. Describe the basic, underlying rhythm first, then add its*

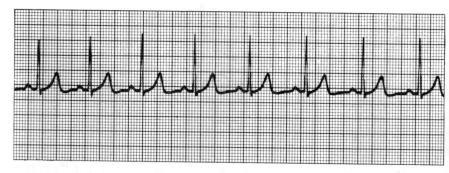

FIGURE 6-1. Normal sinus rhythm. The heart rate is approximately 80 bpm. (Reprinted with permission. Textbook of Advanced Cardiac Life Support, 1987. Copyright American Heart Association.)

*appropriate qualifiers,* such as "sinus rhythm *with* first-degree AV block" or "sinus tachycardia *with* multiform ventricular premature complexes."

# ☐ SINUS TACHYCARDIA

## DEFINITION

Sinus tachycardia (ST) is sinus rhythm at a rate equal to or greater than 100 bpm.

## ETIOLOGY

1. Situations of increased physiologic demand for oxygen that occur in association with stress, exercise, pain, fever, anemia, hypoxia, and shock
2. Hyperthyroidism, heart failure, myocardial infarction, pulmonary embolism, medications (e.g., atropine, epinephrine, isoproterenol), and excessive caffeine
3. Physiologic ST commonly observed in neonates (the heart rate may range between 100 and 160 bpm)

## CHARACTERISTICS

Sinus tachycardia has the same characteristics as NSR, except that in ST the ventricular rate is equal to or greater than 100 bpm. Normally, ST results from a gradual acceleration of sinus node discharge.

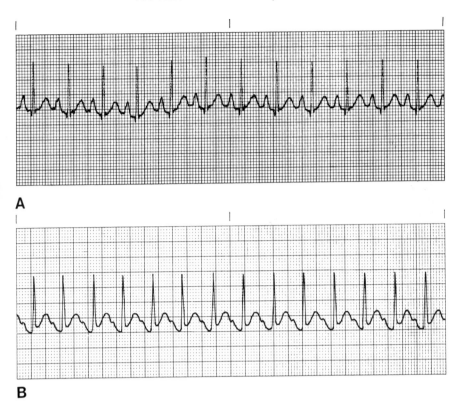

**A**

**B**

**FIGURE 6-2.** Sinus tachycardia. (*A*) The heart rate is approximately 125 bpm. (*B*) The heart rate is approximately 136 bpm. As the rate increases, the P wave gets closer to the preceding T wave. In this example, the P wave actually distorts the downstroke of the T wave. (From Walraven, G: Basic Arrhythmias, ed 2. Brady Publishing, Englewood Cliffs, NJ, 1986, pp 71, 83, with permission.)

## TREATMENT

Sinus tachycardia may be accompanied by rate-related symptoms, especially in patients with underlying heart disease. Shortened diastolic filling time can result in reduced forward stroke volume and may lead to heart failure. Tachycardia also increases myocardial oxygen demand, which may be detrimental in patients with coronary artery disease.

1. Therapy should be guided by evaluating accompanying symptomatology (e.g., dizziness, weakness, anginal pain, hypotension). The tachycardia may subside spontaneously if the underlying cause is treated successfully, thereby negating the need for drug therapy.
2. Consider the use of beta blockers and calcium channel blockers to slow the rate, if necessary, but be aware of the potential side effects of drug

therapy. Specifically, noncardioselective beta blockers (e.g., propranolol) may exacerbate asthma or other pulmonary conditions; calcium channel blockers (e.g., intravenous verapamil) may produce significant hypotension and may also depress the inotropic action of the heart, leading to heart failure.

> ### CLINICAL TIP
>
> By definition, *any* rhythm in which the rate is 100 bpm or greater is classified as **tachycardia.** Patients with normal hearts may tolerate tachycardia quite easily, but those with diseased hearts may be unable to maintain adequate cardiac output.

# ☐ SINUS BRADYCARDIA

## DEFINITION

Sinus bradycardia (SB) is sinus rhythm with a rate less than 60 bpm.

## ETIOLOGY

1. Vagal stimulation, physiologic causes (in well-trained athletes), sleep
2. Hypothyroidism, hypothermia, electrolyte imbalances (e.g., hyperkalemia)
3. Inferior wall myocardial infarction
4. Sick sinus syndrome
5. Medications (e.g., beta blockers, calcium channel blockers, digoxin)

## CHARACTERISTICS

The characteristics for SB are the same as for NSR, except the ventricular rate in SB is slower than 60 bpm.

## TREATMENT

Sinus bradycardia can result in reduced cardiac output and breakthrough dysrhythmias. Treatment is guided by evaluation of the underlying cause and by whether symptoms are present.

1. Drug therapy (including atropine and epinephrine) should be considered for patients who manifest signs of hypoperfusion or are symptomatic (dizzy, weak, or hypotensive).
2. Pacemakers (temporary or permanent) may be required if drug therapy is ineffective.

MCL₁

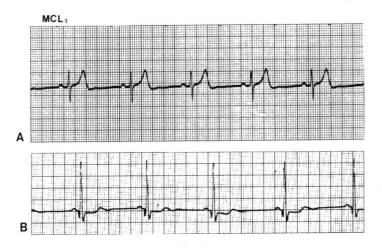

A

B

**FIGURE 6-3.** Sinus bradycardia. *(A)* The heart rate is approximately 56 bpm. (From Brown, KR and Jacobson, S: Mastering Dysrhythmias: A Problem-Solving Guide. FA Davis, Philadelphia, 1988, p 69, with permission.) *(B)* The heart rate is approximately 50 bpm. (From Conover, MB: Understanding Electrocardiography: Arrhythmias and the 12-Lead ECG, ed 5. CV Mosby, St. Louis, 1988, p 86, with permission.)

**CLINICAL TIP**
Atropine is the drug of choice to treat *symptomatic* bradycardia (i.e., slow rate accompanied by weakness, hypotension, anginal pain). Epinephrine may be used if atropine is ineffective.

**CLINICAL TIP**
By definition, *any* rhythm with a rate less than 60 bpm is classified as a **bradycardia.** Patients with normal hearts usually tolerate bradycardia with no ill effects, but, in the presence of a slow rate, patients with diseased hearts may be unable to maintain an adequate cardiac output.

# SINUS ARRHYTHMIA (OR SINUS DYSRHYTHMIA)

## DEFINITION

Sinus arrhythmia is usually a sinus rhythm with a rate that varies with respiration (respiratory sinus arrhythmia). It is usually a benign rhythm dis-

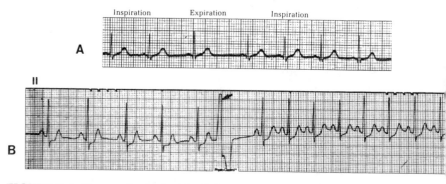

**FIGURE 6-4.** Sinus arrhythmia. The R-R interval is irregular. *(A)* Respiratory sinus arrhythmia. The R-R interval shortens with inspiration and lengthens with expiration. (From Conover, MB: Understanding Electrocardiography: Arrhythmias and the 12-Lead ECG, ed 5. CV Mosby, St. Louis, 1988, p 87, with permission.) *(B)* Nonrespiratory sinus arrhythmia. The irregularity of the R-R interval is not associated with the respiratory cycle. There is one ventricular premature complex *(arrow).* (From Lounsbury, P and Frye, SJ: Cardiac Rhythm Disorders: A Nursing Process Approach, ed 2. Mosby-Year Book, St. Louis, 1992, p 95, with permission.)

turbance characterized by alternate speeding up and slowing down of the heart rate. Rarely, sinus arrhythmia is not associated with respiration (nonrespiratory sinus arrhythmia).

## ETIOLOGY

1. **Respiratory sinus arrhythmia** is a normal finding in children and young adults.
2. **Nonrespiratory sinus arrhythmia** may be observed in persons with cardiac disease and myocardial infarction, especially in association with sinus bradycardia, digoxin therapy, or enhanced vagal tone.

## CHARACTERISTICS

The characteristics of sinus arrhythmia are the same as those for NSR, but in sinus arrhythmia the R-R interval varies.

1. In respiratory sinus arrhythmia, the rate increases with inspiration and decreases with expiration.
2. In nonrespiratory sinus arrhythmia, the irregularity of the rhythm is not correlated with the respiratory cycle.

## TREATMENT

1. Evaluation of underlying cause (especially with nonrespiratory sinus arrhythmia)

# Chapter

# 7

# ATRIAL DYSRHYTHMIAS

## ❏ ATRIAL PREMATURE COMPLEXES

### DEFINITION

An atrial premature complex (APC) results from a premature, ectopic, supraventricular impulse that originates somewhere in the atria outside of the sinoatrial (SA) node. APCs are also called premature atrial complexes (PACs).

### ETIOLOGY

1. Normal finding
2. Stress, caffeine, alcohol
3. Heart failure, myocardial ischemia, valvular diseases, coronary artery disease
4. Chronic lung disease, hyperthyroidism, infection
5. Electrolyte abnormalities (hypokalemia); use of medications (digoxin)

### CHARACTERISTICS

1. The R-R interval is irregular. The premature complex disturbs the regularity of the underlying rhythm.
2. The shape of the ectopic premature P wave is different from the sinus P wave.
3. The premature P wave is followed by a QRS complex if the impulse is conducted into the ventricles.

   **Note:** If the APC occurs so early that the atrioventricular (AV) node has not fully repolarized from the previous impulse, the AV node will be unable to conduct to the ventricles and the premature P wave will

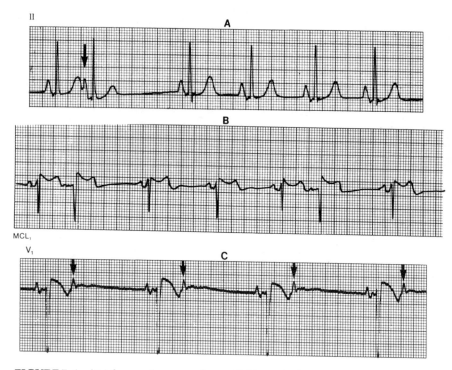

**FIGURE 7-1.** Atrial premature complexes. (*A*) Sinus rhythm with one APC. An ectopic P wave *(arrow)* is clearly visible before the early QRS complex. The QRS is narrow because conduction in the ventricles is undisturbed. (From Conover, MB: Understanding Electrocardiography: Arrhythmias and the 12-Lead ECG, ed 5. CV Mosby, St. Louis, 1988, p 103, with permission.) (*B*) Sinus bradycardia with two APCs (the second and sixth beats). (From Brown, KR and Jacobson, S: Mastering Dysrhythmias: A Problem-Solving Guide. FA Davis, Philadelphia, 1988, p 44, with permission.) (*C*) Sinus rhythm with blocked APCs. Every other P wave is an APC *(arrows)*. The ectopic P wave is premature and is not followed by a QRS complex. (From Lounsbury, P and Frye, SJ: Cardiac Rhythm Disorders. A Nursing Process Approach, ed 2. Mosby-Year Book, Inc., St. Louis, 1992, with permission.)

*not* be followed by a QRS complex. This is known as a **blocked** or **non-conducted APC** and is the most common cause of a pause during sinus rhythm.

4. The QRS complex is narrow if conduction in the ventricles is undisturbed.

**Note:** If the AV node conducts a premature impulse into the ventricles when they have not fully repolarized, the resulting QRS complex may appear wide and abnormally shaped. This is known as an APC conducted with aberration (see p 111) and must be differentiated from a ventricular premature complex (VPC) (see Box 7-1), for both complexes can appear deceptively similar in configuration.

5. The PR interval may be normal, short, prolonged, or absent. The length of the PR interval depends on the ability of the AV node to conduct the early impulse to the ventricles.
6. The APC may occur so early that it distorts the T wave of the previous QRS complex. An abnormal or notched T wave followed by an early QRS complex should always arouse the suspicion of an APC.

**CLINICAL TIP**
The best leads for assessment of atrial rhythm disturbances are II, III, aVF, and V₁ because P waves are usually most prominent in these leads.

## TREATMENT

Therapy for APCs is usually not indicated unless untoward clinical signs and symptoms are present. However, frequent or sustained APCs, if left untreated, may precede other supraventricular dysrhythmias such as atrial fibrillation, so attention should be paid to determining the underlying cause. If drug therapy is recommended, agents such as quinidine, procainamide, and disopyramide may be used.

# ☐ WANDERING ATRIAL PACEMAKER

## DEFINITION

Wandering atrial pacemaker produces a supraventricular rhythm in which pacemaker impulses originate from two or more sites in the SA node, atria, or AV junction and discharge at a rate of 60 to 100 beats per minute (bpm).

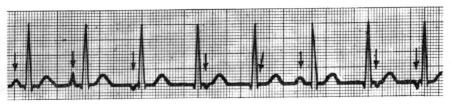

FIGURE 7–2. Wandering atrial pacemaker. The P waves change their shape as the pacemaker "wanders" between sites in the SA node and AV junction. (From Lipman, BC and Lipman, BS: ECG Pocket Guide. Year Book Medical Publishers, Chicago, 1987, p 55, with permission.)

## ETIOLOGY

1. Chronic lung disease
2. Valvular (especially mitral and tricuspid) heart disease

## CHARACTERISTICS

1. P wave morphologies vary because impulses originate from different sites.
2. P-P intervals (and subsequent R-R intervals) may also vary because each impulse travels through the atria via a slightly different route.
3. There is one P wave for every QRS complex.
4. The overall atrial and ventricular rates remain between 60 and 100 bpm.
5. The QRS complexes are usually unchanged. They are narrow as long as ventricular depolarization is undisturbed.

## TREATMENT

Treatment for wandering atrial pacemaker is geared toward resolving the underlying cause.

# ☐ ATRIAL TACHYCARDIA

## DEFINITION

Atrial tachycardia (AT) is a supraventricular rhythm originating in the atria outside of the SA node at a rate between 120 and 250 bpm. Atrial tachycardia is frequently a result of digitalis toxicity.

## ETIOLOGY

1. Digitalis toxicity
2. Valvular (especially rheumatic) heart disease
3. Coronary artery disease
4. Acute myocardial infarction
5. Electrolyte disturbances
6. Idiopathic causes

## CHARACTERISTICS

1. The rhythm is regular (R-R intervals are equal).
2. The atrial rate is 120 to 250 bpm. P-P intervals are equal.
3. Conduction is commonly 1:1 (one P wave for every QRS complex). However, conduction may be 2:1 or greater (two or more P waves for

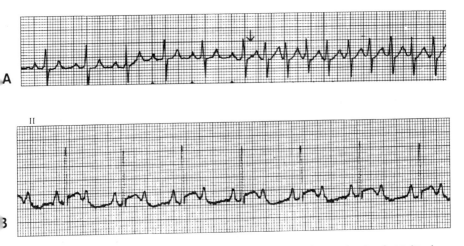

**FIGURE 7-3.** Atrial tachycardia. (*A*) Sinus tachycardia with an episode of atrial tachycardia initiated by an APC *(arrow).* There is 1:1 conduction at a rate of 185 bpm. (Reprinted with permission. Textbook of Advanced Cardiac Life Support, 1987, p70. Copyright American Heart Association.) (*B*) AT with 2:1 AV block caused by digitalis. There are two P waves for every QRS complex. The ventricular rate is approximately half the atrial rate. (From Conover, MB: Understanding Electrocardiography: Arrhythmias and the 12-Lead ECG, ed 5. CV Mosby, St. Louis, 1988, p 108, with permission.)

every QRS complex with an isoelectric baseline between successive P waves), especially in the presence of digitalis toxicity. This phenomenon is sometimes called **atrial tachycardia with AV block.** The abnormal conduction ratios (2:1, 3:1, and so on) that often accompany digitalis toxicity reflect drug-induced conduction block (digitalis inhibits conduction through the AV node) as well as efforts by the AV node to triage the impulses that are bombarding it.

4. The PR interval is short when conduction through the AV node is 1:1. The speed of conduction through the AV node accelerates as the rate increases, thereby shortening the PR interval.
5. P wave morphology is often different from that seen in normal sinus rhythm (NSR). At faster rates, the ectopic P wave may be difficult to see and may distort the T wave of the preceding beat. Leads II, III, aVF, and $V_1$ should be examined carefully for their presence.
6. The shape of the QRS is unchanged from that seen during NSR unless conduction in the ventricles is disturbed.
7. Atrial tachycardia may occur in paroxysms (bursts); when it terminates, there may be a long pause before NSR resumes.

## TREATMENT

1. Withhold digoxin.
2. Treat underlying heart disease.

3. Correct electrolyte abnormalities such as hypokalemia and hypomagnesemia that commonly accompany this dysrhythmia during digitalis toxicity.

 **CLINICAL TIP**

When AT with 2:1 conduction is observed, digitalis toxicity should be the first consideration.

# ☐ MULTIFOCAL ATRIAL TACHYCARDIA

## DEFINITION

Multifocal atrial tachycardia (MAT) is an ectopic supraventricular tachycardia that originates from three or more atrial foci at a rate of 100 to 250 bpm.

## ETIOLOGY

1. Chronic lung disease (especially in the decompensated state)
2. Acute respiratory distress
3. Hypoxemia
4. Pulmonary embolism
5. Pneumonia

## CHARACTERISTICS

1. Three or more P wave configurations (multiple foci)
2. One P wave for every QRS complex (1:1 conduction)
3. Irregular rhythm; varying P-P and R-R intervals
4. PR intervals varying slightly from beat to beat

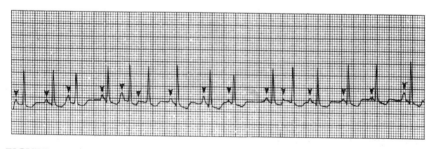

FIGURE 7-4. Multifocal atrial tachycardia. Note the varying P wave morphologies. The PR intervals are variable, and the rhythm is irregular. (From Lipman, BC and Lipman, BS: ECG Pocket Guide. Year Book Medical Publishers, Chicago, 1987, p 56, with permission.)

5. QRS complexes possibly identical to each other or slightly widened secondary to aberrant intraventricular conduction (see p 111)
6. Rate greater than 100 bpm

## TREATMENT

1. Aggressive therapy is directed toward resolution of the underlying cause (most often acute or chronic lung disease).
2. Antidysrhythmic therapy using intravenous (IV) verapamil or metoprolol has been used to slow the heart rate or convert MAT to NSR.

**CLINICAL TIP**
Antidysrhythmic therapy must be used cautiously in patients with preexisting cardiac or pulmonary disease. Verapamil (a calcium channel blocker) may exacerbate heart failure, and metoprolol (a beta blocker) may exacerbate underlying lung disease.

# ☐ PAROXYSMAL SUPRAVENTRICULAR TACHYCARDIA*

## DEFINITION

Paroxysmal supraventricular tachycardia (PSVT) describes two types of rhythm disturbances in which supraventricular impulses are conducted abnormally between the atria and the ventricles. In both forms of PSVT, the ventricles are depolarized at a rate greater than 100 bpm.

## ETIOLOGY

The hallmark of PSVT is abnormal conduction through a **reentry circuit** (or circular conduction pathway), resulting in a rapid supraventricular dysrhythmia. A reentry circuit is formed by two pathways that are connected at their upper and lower ends, providing an uninterrupted circuit for impulse conduction.

In the more common form of PSVT, called **AV nodal reentry tachycardia (AVNRT),** a **microreentry circuit** involving two pathways in the AV junction is implicated. A supraventricular impulse is conducted slowly down one pathway in the AV node toward the ventricles and is then conducted rapidly back into the atria along a second pathway within the AV node. The atria and ventricles are depolarized almost simultaneously. Abnormal conduction is per-

---

*Formerly called paroxysmal atrial tachycardia (PAT).

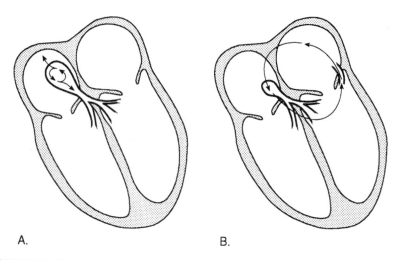

A.                                    B.

**FIGURE 7–5.** Reentry circuits associated with PSVT. (A) A reentry circuit in the AV node comprised of a slow and a fast pathway. The impulse travels into the ventricles via the slow pathway and returns to the atria via the fast pathway. Depolarization of atria and ventricles is almost simultaneous. (B) An accessory bypass tract connecting the atria and ventricles. The impulse travels normally through the AV node into the ventricles and rapidly returns to the atria along the accessory bypass tract. Depolarization of atria and ventricles is sequential.

petuated when the impulse reenters the circuit and travels toward the ventricles again along the same pathway.

The less common form of PSVT, called **atrioventricular reentrant tachycardia (AVRT),** uses a **macroreentry** circuit, called the bundle of Kent, that bypasses the AV node to form an accessory bridge from the atria to the ventricles. AVRT is closely associated with the Wolff-Parkinson-White (WPW) syndrome, a condition discussed more fully in Chapter 15. In the most common form of AVRT (called orthodromic AVRT), supraventricular impulses are conducted normally through the AV node into the ventricles, then quickly reenter the atria by traveling along the accessory bypass tract. The atria and ventricles are depolarized sequentially. As with AVNRT, the cycle in AVRT perpetuates itself as the impulse repeatedly travels the same route.

In **orthodromic AVRT,** impulses are conducted into the ventricles through the AV node and then retrogradely back into the atria along the accessory bypass tract. The most common form of AVRT, this results in a narrow QRS tachycardia.

In **antidromic AVRT,** impulses are conducted abnormally into the ventricles via the accessory bypass tract and then usually retrogradely into the atria through the AV node. Rarely, impulses may be conducted retrogradely into the atria through a second accessory pathway instead of the AV node. Antidromic AVRT is a less common form of AVRT and produces a wide QRS tachycardia that resembles ventricular tachycardia.

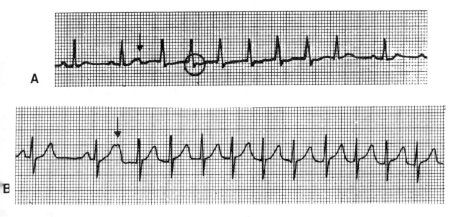

A

E

**FIGURE 7-6.** AV nodal reentry tachycardia. *(A)* Note the long initiating PR interval *(arrow)*; a retrograde P wave distorts the terminal portion of the QRS complex *(circled).* *(B)* The initiating PR interval is long, and the P wave is buried within the QRS complex. (From Conover, MB: Understanding Electrocardiography: Arrhythmias and the 12-Lead ECG, ed 5. CV Mosby, St. Louis, 1988, pp 134, 137, with permission.)

## CHARACTERISTICS

1. An APC usually initiates the reentry process in PSVT.
2. The initiating APC inscribes a P wave followed by a QRS complex (atrioventricular conduction), but subsequent beats reveal either a QRS complex followed by a P wave (ventriculoatrial conduction) or a QRS complex with an imbedded, and therefore invisible, P wave.
3. The QRS complexes in both AVNRT and orthodromic AVRT are normally narrow and regular, but aberrancy (wider than normal QRS complexes) is more common in AVRT because of the increased heart rate.
4. In AVNRT, a retrograde P wave is either buried within the QRS complex or is barely visible, distorting the terminal portion of the QRS. A retrograde P wave is commonly observed following the QRS in AVRT. In both AVNRT and AVRT, retrograde P waves will be negative in the inferior leads (II, III, and aVF).
5. The conduction ratio (ventricular to atrial) is usually 1:1.

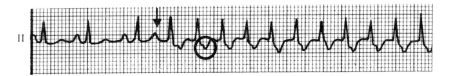

II

**FIGURE 7-7.** Atrioventricular reentry tachycardia. The initiating PR interval is normal, and the retrograde P wave (negative in lead II) is easily visible following the QRS complex. (From Conover, MB: Understanding Electrocardiography: Arrhythmias and the 12-Lead ECG, ed 5. CV Mosby, St. Louis, 1988, p 158, with permission.)

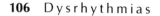

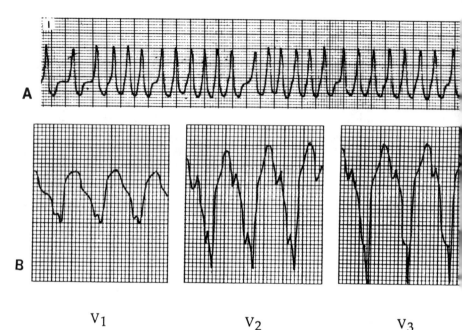

$V_1$ $V_2$ $V_3$

**FIGURE 7-8.** Atrioventricular reentry tachycardia. (A) AVT in a patient with atrial fibrillation and Wolff-Parkinson-White Syndrome. The ventricular rate is approximately 250 bpm. (From Marriott, HJL and Conover, MB: Advanced Concepts in Arrhythmias, ed 2. CV Mosby, St. Louis, 1989, p 165, with permission.) (B) The wide QRS complexes resemble ventricular tachycardia (antidromic AVT).

6. The onset and termination of PSVT is usually abrupt.
7. The ventricular rate is greater than 100 bpm. A rate exceeding 200 bpm suggests AVRT.

## TREATMENT

Choice of therapy is contingent on the type of PSVT present.
**For AVNRT,**

1. Vagal maneuvers (e.g., carotid sinus massage, Valsalva maneuver, immersion of the face in cold water) can be performed.
2. Administer drugs that act directly on the AV node to slow conduction in the anterograde (slow) pathway, including adenosine, calcium channel blockers (e.g., verapamil and diltiazem), beta blockers (e.g., propranolol and metoprolol), and digoxin.
3. If the patient is symptomatic (e.g., hypotensive or in acute distress), synchronized cardioversion using 50 joules (to start) may be performed.
4. For recurrent AVNRT, ablation of the microreentry circuit may be indicated. Chronic drug therapy includes class IA, class IC, and class III antidysrhythmic agents.

## For AVRT

1. Vagal maneuvers
2. Adenosine and beta blockers may be given to slow conduction through the AV node. Calcium Channel blockers and digitalis also may be given cautiously as they may increase conduction through the accessory pathway which can be dangerous if atrial fibrillation develops.

   **Note:** Vagal maneuvers and drugs that block the AV node (adenosine, beta blockers, calcium channel blockers, digitalis) may not be effective in terminating **antidromic AVRT** if the retrograde pathway to the atria is another accessory pathway instead of the AV node.

3. Antidysrhythmic agents that block conduction in the accessory bypass tract (e.g., class I agents, class III agents)
4. Synchronized cardioversion
5. Surgical interruption or ablation of the accessory pathway

**CLINICAL TIP**

The best course of therapy is determined from the results of electrophysiologic studies that show the precise route of impulse transmission. If the patient develops signs or symptoms of hypoperfusion, urgent electrical cardioversion should be performed, regardless of the etiology of the PSVT.

WPW syndrome can be dangerous because of the associated exceedingly fast rates of conduction through the accessory bypass tract. If atrial fibrillation develops in patients with WPW, the extremely fast ventricular rate may degenerate into ventricular fibrillation.

# □ ATRIAL FLUTTER

## DEFINITION

Atrial flutter is a supraventricular dysrhythmia characterized by the appearance of sawtooth-shaped **flutter waves** at a rate between 250 and 350 bpm. Atrial flutter is thought to be associated with a reentry mechanism within the atria (see p 103).

## ETIOLOGY

1. Hyperthyroidism
2. Valvular disease (especially rheumatic mitral stenosis and regurgitation)
3. Ischemic heart disease, acute myocardial infarction
4. Pericardial disease
5. Acute pulmonary embolism

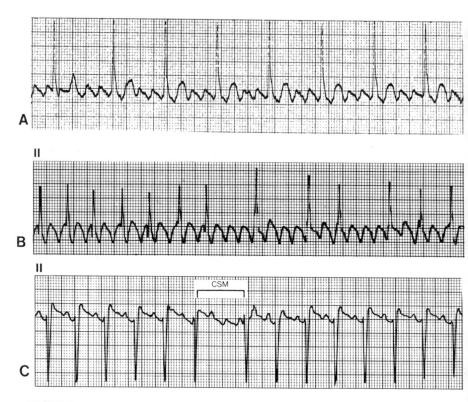

A

II

B

II

C

**FIGURE 7–9.** Atrial flutter. Note the sawtooth shape of the flutter waves. *(A)* Atrial with 4:1 conduction (one of the flutter waves is obscured by the QRS complex). The R-R interval is regular. (From Brown, KR and Jacobson, S: Mastering Dysrhythmias: A Problem-Solving Guide. FA Davis, Philadelphia, 1988, p 221, with permission.) *(B)* Atrial flutter with variable conduction. The R-R interval is irregular. (From Conover, MB: Understanding Electrocardiography: Arrhythmias and the 12-Lead ECG, ed 5. CV Mobsy, St. Louis, 1988, p 117, with permission.) *(C)* Atrial flutter with 2:1 conduction. Carotid sinus massage (CSM) temporarily slows the ventricular rate enough to unmask the flutter waves. (From Brown, KR and Jacobson, S: Mastering Dysrhythmias: A Problem-Solving Guide. FA Davis, Philadelphia, 1988, p 244, with permission.)

6. Pulmonary disease
7. Congenital heart disease
8. Sick sinus syndrome
9. Idiopathic causes

## CHARACTERISTICS

1. P waves are absent. Instead, **flutter** (F) waves represent abnormal depolarization of the atria. They assume a sawtooth or "picket fence" shape that is most easily seen in inferior leads II, III, and aVF, and in precordial lead $V_1$.

2. The F waves appear contiguously with no isoelectric baseline visible between them. Some F waves may be obscured by the QRS complex.
3. The atrial rate (flutter rate) ranges between 250 and 350 bpm (average is 300 bpm).
4. The ventricular rate is usually slower than the atrial rate because the AV node triages impulses (prevents some impulses from conducting to the ventricles). Under normal conditions, the AV node is unable to conduct more than 150 to 200 impulses per minute into the ventricles, especially when drugs (e.g., digitalis) are in the circulatory system.
5. The conduction ratio (ratio of F waves to QRS complexes) is usually an even multiple (2:1, 4:1, 6:1). One-to-one (1:1) conduction is rare.
6. The R-R interval is regular if the conduction ratio is even (e.g., 2:1 or 4:1); it is irregular if the conduction ratio is variable.
7. The QRS complexes are usually narrow as long as conduction in the ventricles is normal.

## TREATMENT

The goal of therapy is to convert atrial flutter to sinus rhythm. This can sometimes be accomplished by correcting the underlying cause. If efforts to convert atrial flutter are unsuccessful, the goal is to maintain control of the ventricular response.

1. Slow the ventricular rate by blocking conduction through the AV node with agents such as digoxin, beta blockers (propranolol or metoprolol), and calcium channel blockers (verapamil or diltiazem).
2. Add class I (quinidine, procainamide, disopyramide), class Ic (flecainide), or class III (amiodarone [for chronic therapy]) antidysrhythmic agents to convert the atrial flutter to sinus rhythm or to slow the firing rate of the ectopic atrial focus.
3. Synchronized cardioversion (starting at 50 joules) should be performed, especially in the presence of hemodynamic compromise.
4. Overdrive pacing may be used to convert atrial flutter to normal sinus rhythm but is not always successful.

### CLINICAL TIP
Flutter waves may be difficult to identify if 2:1 conduction is present. Vagal maneuvers like carotid sinus massage or drugs may be used to increase block at the AV node, thus slowing the ventricular response enough to unmask previously hidden flutter waves. When the vagal maneuver is terminated, the original rapid ventricular rate may return.

### CLINICAL TIP
Atrial flutter can be differentiated from atrial tachycardia by closely examining the baseline. In atrial flutter, F waves are con-

tiguous, whereas in atrial tachycardia, ectopic P waves are separated by an isoelectric baseline.

**CLINICAL TIP**
Cardioversion should be attempted with care in patients taking digoxin. The digitalized heart is very sensitive to electroshock, and ventricular fibrillation or asystole may result when cardioversion is performed. In a nonemergent situation, digitalis may be held temporarily (e.g., for 24 hours) before elective cardioversion.

# ☐ ATRIAL FIBRILLATION

## DEFINITION

Atrial fibrillation is a supraventricular dysrhythmia characterized by multiple ectopic atrial foci, uncoordinated atrial contractions, and a classically irregular ventricular rate. Atrial fibrillation may occur intermittently, (paroxysmal atrial fibrillation), but it frequently becomes a chronic condition.

## ETIOLOGY

1. Heart failure, ischemic heart disease
2. Valvular heart disease (especially mitral stenosis and mitral regurgitation)
3. Cardiomyopathy, alcohol ("holiday heart syndrome"), pericardial disease
4. Congenital heart disease (especially atrial septal defect), WPW syndrome
5. Sick sinus syndrome
6. Hypertension
7. Hyperthyroidism
8. Lung disease (acute and chronic)

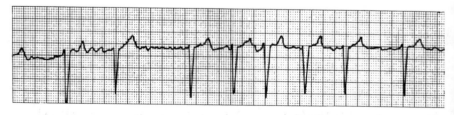

FIGURE 7–10. Atrial fibrillation. Fibrillatory waves distort the baseline, and the R-R interval is characteristically irregular. The ventricular rate is approximately 70 bpm. (Reproduced with permission. Textbook of Advanced Cardiac Life Support, p 73, 1987. Copyright American Heart Association.)

9. Heart surgery
10. Idiopathic causes

## CHARACTERISTICS

1. There are no P waves. Instead, **fibrillatory (f)** waves represent abnormal impulses that arise within the atria. The f waves are small, poorly defined, and distort the baseline; they may be fine or coarse in appearance. If the fibrillatory waves are large, they can be confused with flutter waves, especially in the inferior leads and lead $V_1$. Chaotic atrial depolarization results in uncoordinated mechanical contraction and loss of the "atrial kick." The atrial kick normally provides approximately 20 percent of forward stroke volume.
2. The R-R intervals are irregular because conduction through the AV node is highly variable.
3. QRS complexes are usually narrow unless conduction in the ventricles is abnormal. Because impulses are conducted irregularly through the AV node, the stage is set for aberrant ventricular conduction of some of these impulses. This ECG finding, called Ashman's phenomenon (see Box 7–1), is characterized by wide QRS complexes that can easily be mistaken for ventricular premature complexes (VPCs).

## TREATMENT

The treatment for atrial fibrillation is the same as that for atrial flutter. Overdrive pacing cannot be used for conversion of atrial fibrillation to NSR.

**CLINICAL TIP**
Clots (or thrombi) may form within the atria during atrial fibrillation because of stagnant blood flow. Anticoagulation with heparin or warfarin may have to be considered before and after elective cardioversion. Transesophageal echocardiography may be used to evaluate the presence of left atrial thrombi prior to cardioversion of atrial fibrillation.

---

BOX 7–1 **Aberration—Ashman's Phenomenon**

Aberration (also known as Ashman's phenomenon in the presence of atrial fibrillation) refers to abnormal intraventricular conduction of a supraventricular impulse. The QRS complexes are abnormally wide and may resemble ventricular premature beats.

Normally when a supraventricular impulse reaches the AV node, it is delayed briefly and then travels down both bundle branches essentially

## BOX 7-1 (continued)

at the same time to produce a narrow QRS complex. However, if one of the bundle branches is still refractory (not fully repolarized from the previous beat) when the impulse emerges from the bundle of His, the ventricles will not be depolarized normally. Instead, the impulse will be conducted down the fully recovered branch to depolarize one ventricle in a normal fashion. The impulse will spread abnormally through adjacent muscle cells to depolarize the other ventricle (sequential depolarization). Because total ventricular depolarization takes longer than normal, the resulting QRS complex will appear wider than normal, or aberrant. This QRS resembles a VPC, but it actually originates from a supraventricular site.

Although aberrant QRS complexes are frequently observed during atrial fibrillation, *any* premature supraventricular impulse or sudden rate acceleration can cause aberrant conduction in the ventricles. The danger of aberration lies not in the phenomenon itself but in the *misinterpretation*, which may lead to incorrect treatment. Aberrantly conducted supraventricular impulses are often mistaken for VPCs during atrial fibrillation.

### CLINICAL TIP

Do not fall victim to the "lidocaine reflex"—the tendency to automatically treat a wide QRS complex as ventricular in origin (as a VPC). The abnormal complex may simply represent aberrant conduction.

### CHARACTERISTICS

1. The aberrant complex usually appears when a long cycle length (or R-R interval) is followed by a shorter cycle length. The shorter cycle length terminates with the aberrant complex. This may be referred to as a long-short interval resulting in aberrant conduction.
2. The aberrant QRS complex often assumes an rsR' configuration (like right bundle branch block) in lead $V_1$. This is because the right bundle branch usually takes longer to repolarize than does the left bundle branch.

### TREATMENT

Aberrantly conducted supraventricular complexes require no treatment.

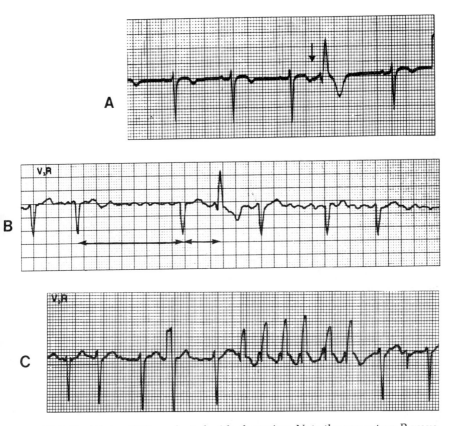

**FIGURE 7–11.** (*A*) An APC conducted with aberration. Note the premature P wave (*arrow*) followed by a QRS complex with an rsR′ configuration. (*B*) Aberration in the presence of atrial fibrillation (the Ashman Phenomenon). A long R-R interval followed by a short R-R interval results in aberrant intraventricular conduction. (*C*) Aberration resembling ventricular tachycardia. The underlying rhythm is atrial fibrillation. A series of aberrantly conducted beats begins after a long-short interval. The R-R interval in this series is irregular, further supporting the diagnosis of aberration. (Reproduced with permission. Textbook of Advanced Cardiac Life Support, p 85, 1987. Copyright American Heart Association.)

# Chapter

# 8

# JUNCTIONAL DYSRHYTHMIAS

## ☐ JUNCTIONAL PREMATURE COMPLEXES

### DEFINITION

A junctional premature complex (JPC) is a premature, ectopic, supraventricular impulse that originates from the area in and around the AV junction. A JPC is also known as a premature junctional complex (PJC).

### ETIOLOGY

1. Normal finding
2. Stress, caffeine, alcohol
3. Heart failure, myocardial ischemia, pericarditis
4. Valvular heart disease, coronary artery disease
5. Chronic lung disease, hyperthyroidism
6. Electrolyte abnormalities (hypokalemia), medications (digoxin)
7. Excessive vagal tone

### CHARACTERISTICS

1. The R-R interval is irregular. The premature complex disturbs the regularity of the underlying rhythm.
2. A visible P wave may or may not be associated with a premature QRS complex. If the P wave is visible, it commonly occurs either just before or just after the QRS complex and is usually inverted in the inferior leads (II, III, aVF). The presence of an inverted P wave implies that the

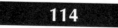

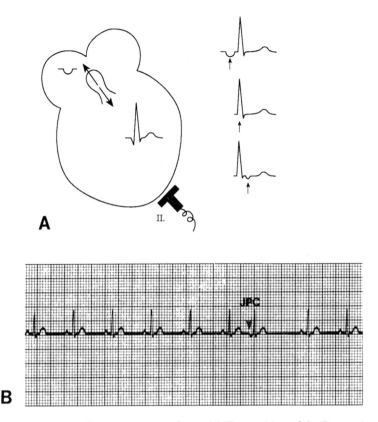

**FIGURE 8-1.** Junctional premature complexes. (A) The position of the P wave in relation to the QRS complex simply indicates which chamber was depolarized first (see text). The P wave may appear before or after the QRS complex, or it may be buried within it. If the P wave is visible, it is usually inverted in the inferior leads. (B) Sinus rhythm with one JPC. Note the inverted P wave (arrow) that appears just before the premature QRS complex. The PR interval is shorter than usual. (From Lipman, BC and Lipman, BS: ECG Pocket Guide. Year Book Medical Publishers, Chicago, 1987, p 54, with permission.)

ectopic impulse from the AV junction was conducted retrogradely (backward) into the atria.

**Note:** The ectopic impulse emerging from the AV junction travels in a retrograde direction to depolarize the atria and in an antegrade direction to depolarize the ventricles. If the P wave appears before the QRS complex, the atria were depolarized before the ventricles. If the P wave occurs immediately after the QRS complex, the atria were depolarized after the ventricles. If the P wave is buried in the QRS complex, it is assumed that the atria and ventricles were depolarized simultaneously.

3. If the premature ectopic P wave precedes the QRS complex, the resulting PR interval is abnormally short—often less than 0.12 second.

4. The QRS complex is narrow as long as intraventricular conduction is undisturbed.

**CLINICAL TIP**

The ectopic P wave associated with a JPC is normally inverted in inferior leads II, III, and aVF. On the other hand, the ectopic P wave associated with an APC may be upright or inverted in these leads, depending on its site of origin. At times it may be impossible to distinguish between the two.

## TREATMENT

Specific therapy for JPCs is usually not indicated. Clinically, JPCs are observed much less frequently than APCs but are associated with similar symptoms.

# ◻ JUNCTIONAL RHYTHM

## DEFINITION

Junctional rhythm is a passive escape rhythm that originates in the AV junction and usually appears secondary to depression of the higher sinus pacemaker.

## ETIOLOGY

1. Acute inferior wall myocardial infarction
2. Heart failure
3. Valvular (especially mitral or tricuspid) heart disease
4. Cardiomyopathy, myocarditis
5. Sick sinus syndrome

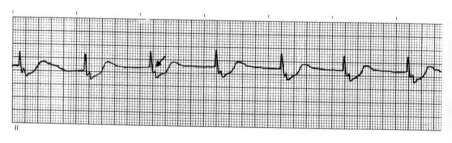

**FIGURE 8–2.** Junctional rhythm. The P wave *(arrow)* appears just after the QRS complex. The R-R interval is regular, and the rate is 60 bpm. (From Brown, KR and Jacobson, S: Mastering Dysrhythmias: A Problem-Solving Guide. FA Davis, Philadelphia, 1988, p 52, with permission.)

6. Drug effects
7. Electrolyte disturbances
8. Normal finding (especially in athletes)

## CHARACTERISTICS

1. The ventricular rate is between 40 and 60 bpm.
2. The R-R interval is regular.
3. There is one P wave for every QRS complex (1:1 conduction). The P wave may appear before the QRS or after the QRS, or it may be buried within the QRS complex.
4. The P wave is usually inverted in the inferior leads (II, III, aVF).
5. If the ectopic P wave precedes the QRS complex, the resultant PR interval is abnormally short—often less than 0.12 second.
6. The QRS complex is narrow as long as intraventricular conduction is undisturbed.

## TREATMENT

1. Determine the underlying cause.
2. Withhold digoxin and any other drugs that may depress the sinus node.
3. If symptoms related to the slow rate are present, efforts to accelerate the sinus pacemaker with drugs such as atropine may be indicated. Artificial pacing may be indicated.

# ☐ ACCELERATED JUNCTIONAL RHYTHM AND JUNCTIONAL TACHYCARDIA

## DEFINITION

Accelerated junctional rhythm and junctional tachycardia represent supraventricular dysrhythmias arising from the AV junction at rates exceeding the inherent junctional escape rate of 40 to 60 bpm.

## ETIOLOGY

1. Digitalis toxicity (often during treatment of atrial fibrillation)
2. Myocardial infarction (especially inferior wall infarction)
3. Acute rheumatic fever
4. Heart failure
5. Valvular heart disease and after cardiac surgery (especially valve surgery)
6. Myocarditis

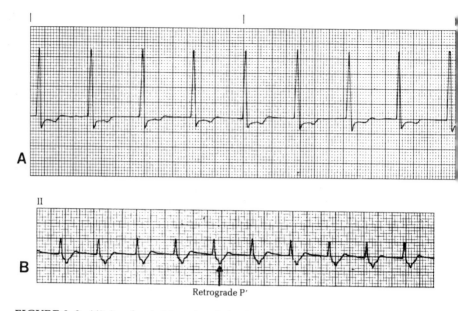

**FIGURE 8-3.** (*A*) Accelerated junctional rhythm. The rhythm is regular, and the rate is approximately 85 bpm. The P wave is buried within the QRS complex. (From Walraven, G: Basic Arrhythmias, ed 2. Brady, Englewood Cliffs, NJ, 1986, p 160, with permission.) (*B*) Junctional tachycardia. The rhythm is regular, and the rate is approximately 110 bpm. A retrograde P wave is visible after each QRS complex. (From Conover, MB: Understanding Electrocardiography: Arrhythmias and the 12-Lead ECG, ed 5. CV Mosby, St. Louis, 1988, p 127, with permission.)

## CHARACTERISTICS

All the characteristics described for junctional escape rhythm apply, except for ventricular rate. In **accelerated junctional rhythm** the ventricular rate is between 60 and 100 bpm. In **junctional tachycardia** the ventricular rate is 100 bpm or faster.

## TREATMENT

1. Investigate the underlying cause, and correct it if possible.
2. If digitalis toxicity is implicated, withhold the drug. Digoxin Immune Fab (digoxin antibodies) may be administered to reverse the toxic effects of digitalis.

### CLINICAL TIP

Both accelerated junctional rhythm and junctional tachycardia may be manifestations of digitalis toxicity, especially during treatment of atrial fibrillation. Digoxin is usually given to slow the characteristically rapid and irregular ventricular response that occurs during atrial fibrillation. If the R-R interval becomes regular in the presence of underlying atrial fibrillation, **complete AV block** with a junctional rhythm should be suspected. It is important to recognize this drug-induced rhythm disturbance because the continued administration of digoxin may precipitate additional, more severe, dysrhythmias.

# Chapter

# 9

# VENTRICULAR DYSRHYTHMIAS

## □ VENTRICULAR PREMATURE COMPLEXES

### DEFINITION

A ventricular premature complex (VPC) is a premature, ectopic impulse that originates somewhere in the ventricles below the bundle of His. VPCs are also called premature ventricular complexes (PVCs).

### ETIOLOGY

1. Normal finding
2. Stress, exercise
3. Excessive intake of caffeine or alcohol
4. Medications (e.g., digoxin or other proarrhythmic drugs)
5. Electrolyte imbalance (e.g., hypokalemia or hypomagnesemia)
6. Coronary artery disease
7. Myocardial ischemia or infarction
8. Cardiomyopathy, pericardial disease
9. Congenital heart disease
10. Hypoxemia, metabolic disorders
11. Reperfusion (e.g., after thrombolytic therapy or angioplasty)
12. Heart surgery or contact of the endocardium with catheters (e.g., pacing catheters or flow-directed pulmonary artery catheters)
13. Idiopathic causes

## CHARACTERISTICS

1. The ectopic QRS complex is earlier than expected (premature).
2. The R-R interval is irregular. The premature QRS interrupts the regularity of the underlying rhythm.
3. The ectopic QRS complex is wider than the normal QRS complexes and its morphology is different from the normal beats. The impulse originates from a focus within the ventricles and spreads through the muscle to depolarize the ventricles sequentially. It takes longer than normal to do this, so the resulting QRS complex is wide.
4. The ST segment and T wave slope in the opposite direction from the ectopic QRS complex. *Because depolarization is abnormal, repolarization is also abnormal.*
5. A P wave is usually not seen preceding the ectopic QRS complex, but an inverted P wave may be visible immediately after the ectopic QRS complex if the impulse travels retrogradely to depolarize the atria.

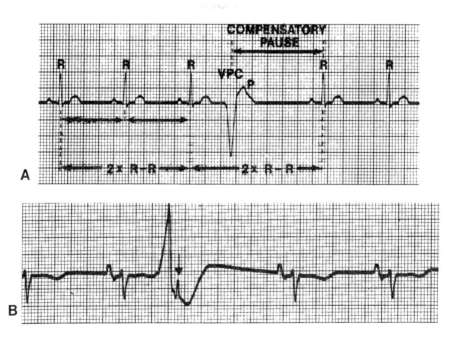

**FIGURE 9–1.** Ventricular premature complexes. (*A*) The ectopic QRS complex (the VPC) is wide, abnormally shaped, and appears earlier than expected. The length of the compensatory pause following the VPC indicates that sinus node discharge was undisturbed (see text). A nonconducted sinus P wave distorts the T wave (the P wave appears on time). (From Lipman, BC and Lipman, BS: ECG Pocket Guide. Year Book Medical Publishers, 1987, p 62, with permission.) (*B*) The P wave immediately following the VPC (*arrow*) indicates that the ectopic impulse was conducted retrogradely into the atria. (From Conover, MB: Understanding Electrocardiography: Arrhythmias and the 12-Lead ECG, ed 5. CV Mosby, St. Louis, 1988, p 187, with permission.)

Sometimes a nonconducted sinus P wave will distort the T wave of the ectopic QRS complex.

6. A long interval of time observed between the VPC and the next normally conducted beat is called a **compensatory pause.** It is assessed by measuring the distance between the two normally conducted sinus beats that surround the VPC and comparing it with the baseline R-R interval.

   - A compensatory pause is commonly observed because the ventricular ectopic impulse traveling retrogradely fails to reach the sinoatrial (SA) node. Sinus discharge remains undisturbed, and the basic underlying sinus rhythm is preserved. The distance between the two normal beats that surround the VPC is two times the baseline R-R interval.
   - Less often, the sinus node is prematurely depolarized by the ventricular ectopic impulse, the SA node resets itself, and no compensatory pause is observed on the ECG. The measured interval is less than two times the baseline R-R interval.

## VARIANTS OF VPCS

- **End-diastolic VPC.** A normal P wave that occurs on time is observed just before the slightly premature ectopic QRS complex. This late-occurring VPC fires after the atria have been depolarized by the sinus impulse but before the sinus impulse reaches the ventricles.
- **Fusion (Dressler) beats.** A VPC fires at the same time that a normally conducted QRS complex occurs. Fusion results when a supraventricular impulse begins to depolarize the ventricles at the same time that an ectopic ventricular impulse starts to do the same thing. Both impulses are responsible for depolarizing a portion of ventricular muscle. The resulting QRS complex represents a blend, or fusing, of normal and ectopic QRS morphologies. Fusion beats are usually wider than normal sinus beats but narrower than VPCs, and their morphologies are highly variable.
- **Interpolated VPC.** A VPC is sandwiched between two normal sinus beats and does not significantly interrupt the underlying rhythm.
- **R-on-T phenomenon.** A VPC occurs on or near the peak of a previous T wave. This is the vulnerable period during ventricular repolarization when VPCs may predispose to ventricular tachycardia or ventricular fibrillation.
- **Uniform VPCs (also called unifocal VPCs).** These VPCs are identical in shape and originate from a single ectopic focus.
- **Multiform VPCs (sometimes called multifocal VPCs).** These VPCs look different *in the same ECG lead.* They usually originate from different ectopic sites, but sometimes they fire from a single site and are conducted along different routes in the ventricles.
- **Couplet.** A couplet is two VPCs (uniform or multiform) in a row.

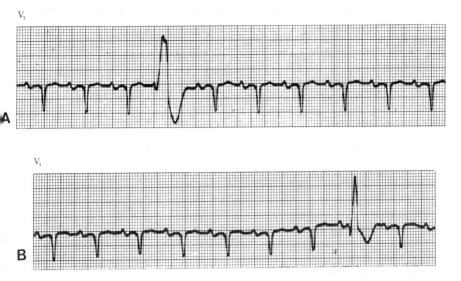

**FIGURE 9-2.** End-diastolic VPCs and fusion beats. (A) End-diastolic VPC. The P wave preceding the VPC comes "on time," and the ectopic QRS complex follows immediately. The VPC is only slightly premature. (B) Fusion beat. The P wave preceding the abnormal QRS complex comes "on time." The QRS complex that follows represents a blending of normal and ectopic morphologies. (From Conover, MB: Understanding Electrocardiography: Arrhythmias and the 12-Lead ECG, ed 5. CV Mosby, St. Louis, 1988, pp 184, 185, with permission.)

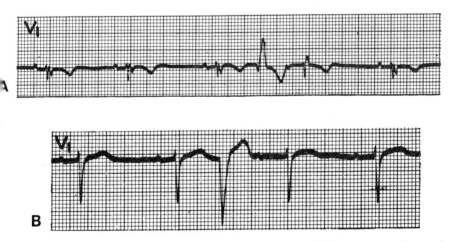

**FIGURE 9-3.** Interpolated VPCs. In both (A) and (B), the VPC appears sandwiched between two sinus beats and does not significantly interrupt the underlying rhythm. (From Marriott, HJL: Practical Electrocardiography, ed 7. Williams & Wilkins, Baltimore, 1983, pp 130, 137, with permission.)

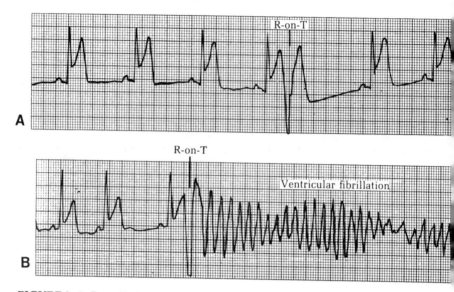

**FIGURE 9-4.** R-on-T phenomenon. (*A*) A VPC occurs near the apex of the T wave. (*B*) A VPC occurs just a little earlier, initiating ventricular fibrillation. (From Conover, MB: Understanding Electrocardiography: Arrhythmias and the 12-Lead ECG, ed 5. CV Mosby, St. Louis, 1988, p 195, with permission.)

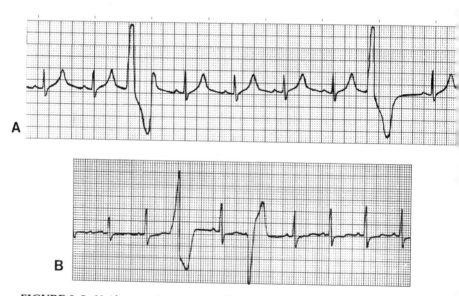

**FIGURE 9-5.** Uniform and multiform VPCs. (*A*) The VPCs assume identical shapes. (From Brown, KR and Jacobson, S: Mastering Dysrhythmias: A Problem-Solving Guide. FA Davis, Philadelphia, p 259, with permission.) (*B*) The VPCs assume different shapes. (Reproduced with permission. Textbook of Advanced Cardiac Life Support, 1987, p 75. Copyright American Heart Association.)

- **Triplet.** A triplet is three VPCs (uniform or multiform) in a row. By definition, three or more consecutive VPCs is termed ventricular tachycardia.
- **Bigeminy.** A uniform VPC alternates with a normal beat in a repeating pattern; every other beat is a VPC. It may be observed in situations of digitalis toxicity. The VPC is coupled or associated with each preceding normal sinus beat. The interval between the VPC and preceding sinus beat is called the coupling interval.
- **Trigeminy.** A uniform VPC alternates with two normal beats in a repeating pattern; every third beat is a VPC.
- **Quadrigeminy.** A uniform VPC alternates with three normal beats in a repeating pattern; every fourth beat is a VPC.
- **Ventricular parasystole.** In ventricular parasystole, an independent ectopic ventricular rhythm is not associated with the underlying sinus rhythm. Ectopic QRS complexes occur at fixed intervals or multiples of a common denominator. Criteria for ventricular parasystole include the following:

   1. The distance between any two ectopic beats (the interectopic interval) is a multiple of the shortest distance between two ectopic beats.
   2. Coupling intervals between ectopic and normal beats vary.
   3. Fusion (Dressler) beats are occasionally found.

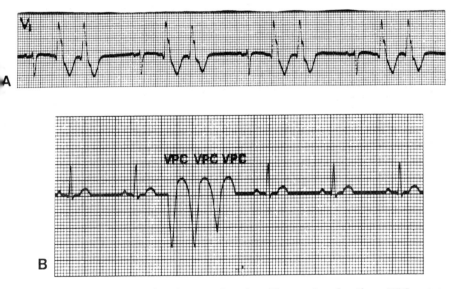

**FIGURE 9-6.** Couplets and triplets. (*A*) Couplets. These pairs of uniform VPCs originate from the same ectopic site. (From Marriott, HJL: Practical Electrocardiography, ed 7. Williams & Wilkins, Baltimore, 1983, p 134, with permission.) (*B*) Triplet. There are three VPCs in a row (technically, this is ventricular tachycardia). (From Lipman, BC and Lipman, BS: ECG Pocket Guide. Year Book Medical Publishers, Chicago, 1987, p 65, with permission.)

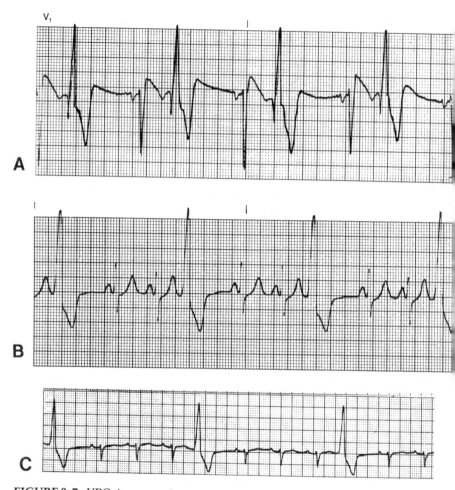

**FIGURE 9-7.** VPCs in a repeating pattern. (*A*) Bigeminy. Every other complex is a uniform VPC. (From Lounsbury, P and Frye, SJ: Cardiac Rhythm Disorders. A Nursing Process Approach, ed 2. Mosby-Year Book, St. Louis, 1992, with permission.) (*B*) Trigeminy. Every third complex is a uniform VPC. (From Walraven, G: Basic Arrhythmias, ed 2. Brady, Englewood Cliffs, NJ, 1986, p 350, with permission.) (*C*) Quadrigeminy. Every fourth complex is a uniform VPC. (From Chung, EK: Electrocardiography: Practical Applications with Vectorial Principles, ed. 3. Appleton & Lange, Norwalk, CT, 1985, p 248, with permission.)

## TREATMENT

Treatment of VPCs should be guided by the clinical setting. Because occasional VPCs are a normal finding in healthy persons, no treatment may be indicated. In addition, if the underlying cause is corrected, VPCs may disappear without specific antidysrhythmic drug therapy. Possible indications for

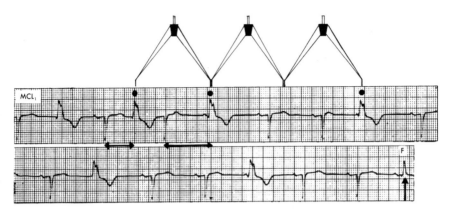

**FIGURE 9-8.** Ventricular parasystole. The longest interectopic interval is twice the shortest interectopic interval (refer to dots above the last three ectopics in the top strip). The coupling intervals vary *(horizontal arrows);* one fusion beat is visible *(vertical arrow).* (Adapted from Marriott, HJL and Conover, MB: Advanced Concepts in Arrhythmias, ed 2. CV Mosby, St. Louis, 1989, p 300, with permission.)

treating VPCs include acute myocardial infarction, cardiomyopathy, structural heart disease, as well as symptoms of palpitations or syncope. The ultimate decision to treat VPCs may require further evaluation such as electrophysiologic study.

Therapeutic options include:

1. Administer antidysrhythmic drugs. In the acute setting, intravenous (IV) drugs such as xylocaine or procainamide may be used. If oral therapy is indicated, agents such as quinidine, procainamide, disopyramide or other antidysrhythmic agents may be given. VPCs resistant to conventional drug treatment may require further evaluation, depending on the clinical setting.

2. Correct underlying electrolyte abnormalities (e.g., hypokalemia).

   **Note.** Electrolyte disturbances are common after surgery.

3. Administer oxygen.

4. Administer magnesium.

**CLINICAL TIP**

Some antidysrhythmic drugs can cause (or worsen) the same dysrhythmias that they are supposed to abolish. These drugs are called **proarrhythmic.** Some antidysrhythmic drugs also depress myocardial function. These potential untoward effects of therapy should always be considered before drugs are administered.

# ☐ IDIOVENTRICULAR RHYTHM

## DEFINITION

An idioventricular rhythm (IVR) is a very slow escape rhythm originating in the ventricles at a rate of 15 to 40 beats per minute (bpm). The appearance of this escape pacemaker occurs when the higher SA nodal or atrioventricular (AV) junctional pacemakers are dysfunctional.

## ETIOLOGY

1. Acute myocardial infarction
2. Cardiomyopathy
3. Myocarditis
4. Drugs (e.g., digitalis)
5. Trauma
6. Dying heart

## CHARACTERISTICS

1. The R-R interval is regular.
2. The ventricular rate is between 15 and 40 bpm.
3. The QRS complexes are wide, and they all look alike.
4. P waves may or may not be present. The absence of P waves suggests that the higher pacemakers are not firing. The presence of upright, normal P waves implies that supraventricular impulses are unable to pen-

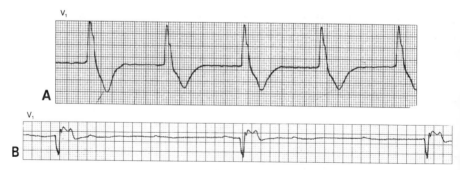

FIGURE 9-9. Idioventricular rhythm. This escape rhythm is slow and regular; the QRS complexes look alike. (*A*) The ventricular rate is approximately 40 bpm. (*B*) The ventricular rate is approximately 15 bpm. P waves appears regularly and are unrelated to the QRS complexes. (From Lounsbury, P and Frye, SJ: Cardiac Rhythm Disorders. A Nursing Process Approach, ed 2. Mosby-Year Book, St. Louis, 1992, with permission.)

etrate the ventricles (see third-degree AV block, p 156). The P-P interval is regular, the P wave rate is faster than the QRS rate, and the P waves are unrelated to the QRS complexes.

## TREATMENT

IVR can cause symptoms such as dizziness, lightheadedness, and syncope because of the slow rate.

1. Correct the underlying cause.
2. Increase the ventricular rate. Atropine is the drug of choice for symptomatic bradycardia, but it may be ineffective if the underlying mechanism is complete heart block.
3. Temporary pacing may be necessary, depending on the clinical situation.
4. Permanent pacing may be indicated.

## CLINICAL TIP
Avoid administration of xylocaine in the presence of an escape rhythm.

# ☐ ACCELERATED IDIOVENTRICULAR RHYTHM

## DEFINITION

Accelerated idioventricular rhythm (AIVR) is an ectopic ventricular rhythm with a rate of 40 to 100 bpm—faster than the normal ventricular escape pacemaker (15 to 40 bpm) but slower than ventricular tachycardia (more than 100 bpm). Its resemblance to ventricular tachycardia has prompted some to describe AIVR using the term "slow ventricular tachycardia."

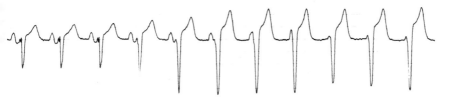

**FIGURE 9–10.** Accelerated idioventricular rhythm. The underlying rhythm is sinus, which is overtaken by AIVR. The QRS complexes are wide, the R-R interval is regular, and the ventricular rate is approximately 90 to 95 bpm.

## ETIOLOGY

1. Acute myocardial infarction (especially inferior wall myocardial infarction)
2. Reperfusion, often after thrombolytic therapy or angioplasty
3. Cardiomyopathy

## CHARACTERISTICS

1. The QRS complexes are wide.
2. The ventricular rate is between 40 and 100 bpm.
3. Ventricular fusion beats often herald the onset and termination of AIVR.
4. Once AIVR is established, the rate may remain regular or gradually decrease.
5. Brief episodes of AIVR may alternate with periods of normal sinus rhythm (NSR), but AIVR may also persist for several minutes at a time.

## TREATMENT

Treatment is usually not required because this benign dysrhythmia is rarely associated with untoward symptoms. However, if the AIVR is slow enough to cause hemodynamic compromise, attempts should be made to accelerate sinus discharge, thereby abolishing the AIVR. Atropine or temporary pacing may be cautiously used to increase the heart rate.

**CLINICAL TIP**
Treatment of AIVR with antidysrhythmic drugs such as xylocaine is *not* recommended. Furthermore, acceleration of the underlying sinus rate should be undertaken cautiously, especially in the setting of acute myocardial infarction. "Tincture of time" is most often the best remedy.

**CLINICAL TIP**
If AIVR degenerates into ventricular tachycardia, treatment with conventional antidysrhythmic drugs and/or cardioversion should be undertaken without delay.

# □ VENTRICULAR TACHYCARDIA

## DEFINITION

Ventricular tachycardia (VT) is a rapid ventricular dysrhythmia usually associated with dramatic clinical signs and symptoms. If left untreated, VT may degenerate into fatal ventricular fibrillation.

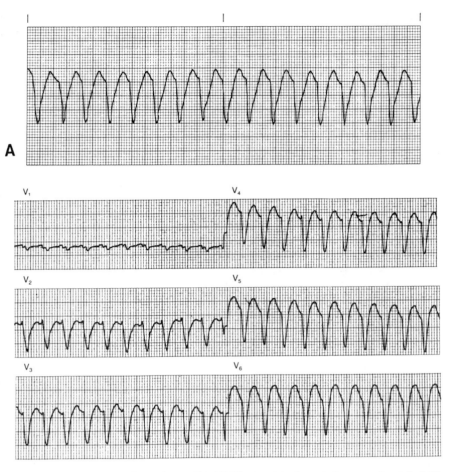

**FIGURE 9-11.** Ventricular tachycardia. (*A*) The ventricular rate is approximately 167 bpm. The QRS complexes are wide, they look alike, and the R-R interval is regular. (From Walraven, G: Basic Arrhythmias, ed 2. Brady, Englewood Cliffs, NJ, 1986, p 282, with permission.) (*B*) The QRS complexes are negative in all six precordial leads. (From Lounsbury, P and Frye, SJ: Cardiac Rhythm Disorders. A Nursing Process Approach, ed 2. Mosby-Year Book, St. Louis, 1992, with permission.)

# ETIOLOGY

1. Acute myocardial ischemia or infarction
2. Cardiomyopathy (ischemic or idiopathic)
3. Myocarditis
4. Electrolyte abnormalities (especially hypokalemia and hypomagnesemia)
5. Medications (e.g., digitalis and proarrhythmic drugs)

6. Mechanical stimulation of the endocardium (e.g., in association with insertion of a pacing catheter or a flow-directed pulmonary artery catheter)
7. Reperfusion
8. Ventricular aneurysm
9. Idiopathic and miscellaneous causes such as right ventricular dysplasia, sarcoidosis, etc.

## CHARACTERISTICS

1. The QRS complexes are usually wider than normal (wide QRS tachycardia).
2. The QRS complexes usually look alike.
3. There are at least three ventricular ectopic beats in a row.
4. The rate is equal to or greater than 100 bpm.
5. The R-R interval is nearly regular.
6. Independent P waves unrelated to the ectopic QRS complexes may appear sporadically (reflecting AV dissociation, a condition characterized by two independent pacemakers). If ventriculoatrial conduction (conduction backward from the ventricles to the atria) is intact, an inverted, retrograde P wave may be visible following each QRS complex.
7. Fusion (Dressler) beats appear if ventricular depolarization results from both sinus and ectopic stimulation; the morphology of the fusion complex reflects a blending of normal and abnormal QRS complexes.
8. Occasionally, sinus impulses are conducted normally into the ventricles during VT. These normally conducted QRS complexes are called **sinus capture beats.**
9. The QRS complexes in the chest leads $V_1$ through $V_6$ are sometimes either all positive or all negative in the presence of VT.

## TREATMENT

Treatment of VT depends on the clinical setting and the ability of the patient to tolerate the dysrhythmia.

1. *Check the pulse.* If there is no pulse (pulseless VT), treat as for ventricular fibrillation (see p 142).
2. If there is a pulse, *evaluate vital signs and clinical symptoms.*
   a. If the patient is tolerating the rhythm (conscious, acceptable vital parameters, no complaints of anginal pain), proceed with drug therapy.
      - Give IV xylocaine, procainamide, or bretylium.
      - If unresponsive to drug therapy, sedate the patient and perform cardioversion, starting at 100 joules; increase as required.

b. If the patient is *not* tolerating the rhythm (unconscious, hypotensive, complaining of anginal pain), attempt to convert the rhythm with a single precordial thump (only if the onset of VT is witnessed in a monitored patient), then proceed immediately with defibrillation.

- Defibrillate at *100 joules initially* (check the ECG after each defibrillation attempt). Unless contraindicated because of hemodynamic deterioration, sedate the patient first.
- Begin drug therapy with xylocaine or bretylium.

Treatment of chronic, recurrent VT includes therapy with oral antidysrhythmic drugs. Further evaluation may include specialized electrophysiologic testing and endocardial mapping. Long-term treatment options for recurrent VT include use of the implantable cardioverter defibrillator (ICD), catheter ablation, and surgery (e.g., cryosurgery, aneurysmectomy).

**CLINICAL TIP**

VT occurring in short bursts (or paroxysms) lasting less than 30 seconds is called **nonsustained VT;** it may cause symptoms such as lightheadedness or anginal pain. Ventricular tachycardia lasting longer than 30 seconds (**sustained VT**) may cause weakness or syncope and may degenerate into ventricular fibrillation.

**CLINICAL TIP**

**Cardioversion** implies application of a *synchronized* electrical shock delivered precisely on the R wave. This is possible only if the ECG signal is transmitted to the cardioverter so that R-wave sensing can occur. **Defibrillation** implies application of an *unsynchronized* electrical shock. The current is delivered randomly during the cardiac cycle. No ECG signal is required for defibrillation.

**CLINICAL TIP**

Whenever electrical shock is required, use safety precautions to prevent patient and/or operator injury.

1. Put the siderails down.
2. Use a conducting medium between the paddles and the skin (defibrillator pads or ECG gel).

---

BOX 9–1 **Ventricular Dysrhythmias Differentiated According to Rate**

| Dysrhythmia | Rate |
| --- | --- |
| VT | 100+ |
| AIVR | 40–100 |
| IVR | 15–40 |

3. Avoid placing the paddles over ECG lead wires, monitoring electrodes, or nitroglycerin patches.
4. Do not charge the machine until you are ready to shock.
5. Perform a last-second *rhythm* check before delivering the shock.
6. Make sure everyone is clear before discharging the paddles.

---

BOX 9–2 **Differentiating the Wide-QRS Tachycardias**

It is tempting to apply the label "ventricular tachycardia" to *all* fast ECG rhythms with a wide QRS complex, but do not be fooled. Diagnosis of wide-QRS tachycardias is not always a sure thing. Wide does *not* automatically imply ventricular.

When a wide-QRS tachycardia originates within the ventricles, the label "VT" is correct. However, wide QRS complexes can also result if supraventricular impulses are conducted abnormally (aberrantly) within the ventricles (as in aberrancy, bundle branch block, and preexcitation). So how does one differentiate between a wide-QRS tachycardia of ventricular origin and one of supraventricular origin?

Knowledge of cardiac history, as well as the availability of old tracings, can be quite helpful. VT is more likely in patients with a previous history of cardiac disease, whereas supraventricular tachycardia is more common in those whose cardiac history is unremarkable or in whom there is evidence of preexisting bundle branch block or preexcitation.

The following criteria are helpful in differentiating **ventricular tachycardia** from **supraventricular tachycardia (SVT) conducted with aberration.** Use limb leads to determine QRS axis, and use the precordial leads to examine QRS morphology.

*Findings Suggestive of Ventricular Tachycardia*

1. QRS duration greater than 0.14 second
2. Left axis deviation (LAD) between $-90°$ and $-180°$ ("no man's land")
3. AV dissociation

   **Note:** Occasional fusion beats or sinus capture beats may be visible.

4. Regular R-R interval
5. Precordial concordance (precordial leads either all positive or all negative)
6. Positive QRS in $V_1$ (or $V_2$)

   • Monophasic or diphasic QRS in $V_1$
   • RSr′ morphology in $V_1$ (left peak taller than right peak)
   • S wave is deeper than the R wave is tall in $V_6$
   • LAD greater than $-30°$ or right axis deviation (RAD) greater than $+120°$

BOX 9-2 (continued)

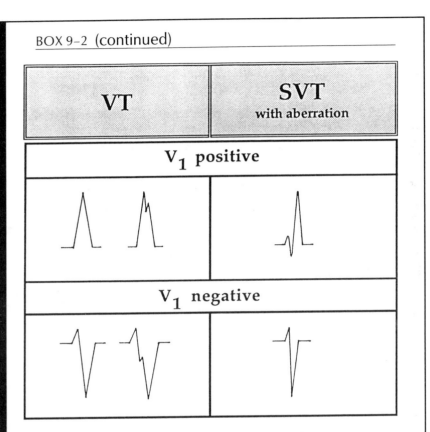

| VT | SVT with aberration |
|---|---|
| $V_1$ positive | |
| $V_1$ negative | |

Differentiating the wide QRS tachycardias.

7. Negative QRS in $V_1$ (or $V_2$)

- R wave greater than 0.04 second
- Slurred downstroke of S wave in $V_1$
- Any Q wave in $V_6$
- Greater than 0.07 second from onset of the QRS to its most negative point in $V_1$

**Findings Suggestive of SVT with Aberration**

1. QRS duration less than 0.14 second
2. Irregular R-R interval
3. Positive QRS in $V_1$ (or $V_2$)

- Triphasic QRS typical of right bundle branch block (RBBB) aberration (rSR')

4. Negative QRS in $V_1$ (or $V_2$)

- QRS typical of left bundle branch block (LBBB) aberration (rS)

---

BOX 9–2 (continued)

- Narrow r (if present)
- Sharp downstroke of S wave

5. Initial portion of the QRS resembles the normal QRS

**If** the origin of a wide QRS tachycardia is not clear, assess the patient's tolerance of the rhythm before rushing to intervene.

Hemodynamically compromised? Perform cardioversion at once.

Consider IV procainamide or adenosine administration.

- Procainamide may convert both VT and SVT
- Adenosine may convert SVT; it is ultrashort-acting (success will be apparent within seconds)

Avoid administration of IV verapamil.

- Can cause profound hemodynamic deterioration if VT present

---

# ☐ VENTRICULAR FLUTTER

## DEFINITION

Ventricular flutter is ventricular rhythm that looks like a very rapid VT. Ventricular flutter is often a precursor to ventricular fibrillation.

## ETIOLOGY

Ventricular flutter has the same etiology as VT.

## CHARACTERISTICS

1. The rate is between 250 and 300 bpm.
2. Discrete QRS complexes as well as ST-segment and T-wave deflections are difficult to visualize. Large-amplitude waveforms appear contiguously (no baseline is visible between them).

## TREATMENT

Ventricular flutter is so rapid that cardiac output is quickly compromised. The result is acute cardiovascular collapse and cardiac arrest.

1. Urgent defibrillation is the treatment of choice. Synchronized cardioversion should not be attempted because the cardioverter, unable to distinguish an R wave, will not fire.

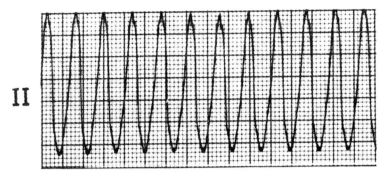

**FIGURE 9–12.** Ventricular flutter. The ventricular rate is approximately 215 bpm. Discrete QRS complexes are hard to identify. (From Chung, EK: Electrocardiography: Practical Applications with Vectorial Principles, ed 3. Appleton & Lange, Norwalk, CT, 1985, p 264, with permission.)

2. Administer antidysrhythmic drugs such as xylocaine and procainamide.
3. Perform cardiopulmonary resuscitation (CPR).

# ☐ TORSADE DE POINTES

## DEFINITION

Torsade de pointes (TdP) is a unique variant of VT in which the QRS complexes appear to twist around the baseline. Torsade de pointes is frequently found with abnormal prolongation of the QT interval. Though often self-limiting, this dysrhythmia can degenerate into ventricular fibrillation.

## ETIOLOGY

1. Class IA antidysrhythmic drugs (quinidine, procainamide, and disopyramide) and class III antidysrhythmic drugs (such as amiodarone and sotolol)
2. Electrolyte abnormalities (especially hypomagnesemia, hypokalemia, and hypocalcemia)
3. Psychotropic drugs
4. Liquid protein diets
5. Romano-Ward syndrome, Jervell-Lange-Nielsen syndrome, and other congenital disorders which cause a prolonged QT interval
6. Acute myocardial infarction

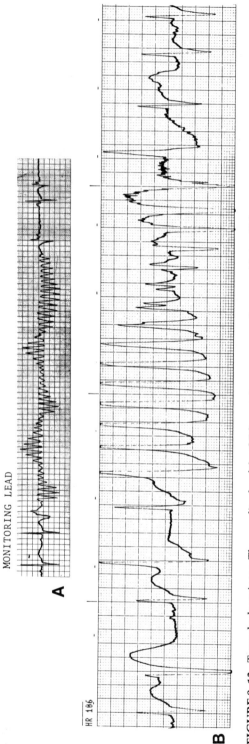

MONITORING LEAD

A

HR 106

B

**FIGURE 9–13.** Torsade de pointes. The amplitude of the QRS complexes waxes and wanes. (*A*) A self-limiting episode of TdP. (From Arcebal, AG and Lemberg, L: Torsade de pointes. Heart Lung 9: 1096, 1980, with permission.) (*B*) This example was obtained from Bernard S. Lipman, MD, as a patient who was receiving quinidine at the time.

## CHARACTERISTICS

1. The polarity of the QRS complexes alternate around the baseline. TdP was originally described by Dessertenne as "twisting of the points."
2. The amplitude of the QRS complexes waxes and wanes.
3. The ventricular rate is extremely rapid.

## TREATMENT

1. Discontinue or withhold the offending antidysrhythmic agents.
2. Correct electrolyte abnormalities.
3. Consider magnesium, xylocaine, isoproterenol, phenytoin, or overdrive pacing to increase heart rate in the acute situation.
4. Perform cardioversion if sustained.
5. Chronic therapy includes beta blockers, pacemaker, ICD implantation, or upper left thoracic sympathectomy.

### CLINICAL TIP
Monitor QT intervals and electrolyte levels in all patients receiving class IA and class III antidysrhythmic agents.

# VENTRICULAR FIBRILLATION

## DEFINITION

Ventricular fibrillation (VF) is a catastrophic dysrhythmia characterized by total disorganization of electrical activity in the heart. In the absence of ECG monitoring, VF cannot be distinguished from ventricular asystole because both rhythms result in clinical cardiac arrest (no cardiac pumping, resulting in loss of pulse and blood pressure).

## ETIOLOGY

1. Myocardial ischemia (e.g., as with acute myocardial infarction)
2. Cardiomyopathy
3. Electrolyte abnormalities (as in VT)
4. Drug toxicity (especially digitalis and prodysrhythmic agents)
5. Failure to synchronize properly during cardioversion
6. Accidental electrical shock (e.g., current leakage from improperly grounded electrical equipment, lightning injury)

## CHARACTERISTICS

1. VF has no identifiable ECG waveforms.
2. Undulating, wavy baseline is composed of waveforms that vary in amplitude and morphology. Early in the course of VF, these fibrillatory

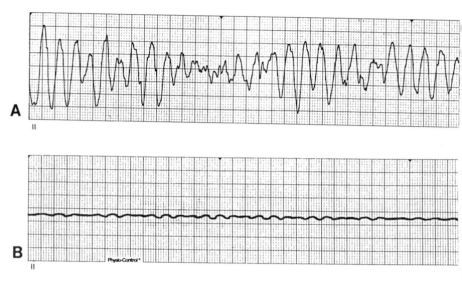

**FIGURE 9-14.** Ventricular fibrillation. There are no identifiable waveforms, and the baseline appears to undulate. (*A*) Coarse VF. (*B*) Fine VF. (From Brown, KR and Jacobson, S: Mastering Dysrhythmias: A Problem-Solving Guide. FA Davis, Philadelphia, 1988, pp 125, 128, with permission.)

waveforms are exaggerated, and the rhythm is described as "coarse VF." After several minutes of ventricular fibrillation, the fibrillatory waveforms become smaller and smaller, and the rhythm is described as "fine VF."

### CLINICAL TIP

Fine VF may resemble ventricular asystole. Confirm your impression by examining the rhythm in different leads.

---

### BOX 9-3 **Automated External Defibrillation**

Automated external defibrillators (AEDs) represent an advance in defibrillator technology. AEDs analyze cardiac electrical activity and deliver programmed electric shocks through large adhesive pads attached to the victim's anterior chest. They are primarily designed for use by first responders in the field but may also be used in hospital or clinic settings whenever access to traditional advanced life support equipment and personnel is delayed.

The primary reason for AED use is to improve survival in cardiac arrest victims. VT (the most common initiating dysrhythmia) deteriorates rapidly to VF—and may progress to irreversible asystole—so *early* defibrillation is considered a critical link in the American Heart Association

## BOX 9-3 (continued)

(AHA) "chain of survival." Prompt application of AED technology may save precious minutes. The first responder with access to an AED applies large pads to the anterior chest wall that are connected via a cable system to the system analyzer. *Fully automated* AEDs analyze the cardiac rhythm and deliver a shock if a nonperfusing dysrhythmia such as VF or VT is present. The operator is not required to interpret the rhythm or to initiate any commands. *Semiautomated* AEDs work in much the same way except that rhythm analysis and delivery of the electric shocks are under operator control.

AEDs are safe and simple to operate, but they must not be used unless the victim is apneic and pulseless. Clearly, accurate initial assessment of clinical status is essential to guarantee the appropriate application of this new technology. For further information about AEDs, the reader should refer to sources such as the AHA's *Manual for Advanced Cardiac Life Support.*

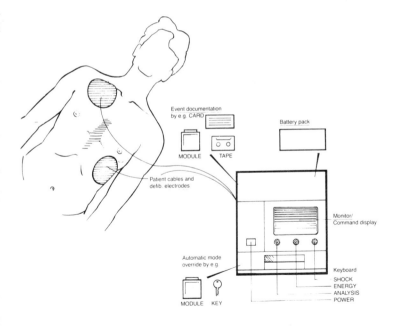

Automated external defibrillation. Schematic of AED attachments. (Reprinted with permission. Textbook of Advanced Cardiac Life Support, 1987, p 290. Copyright American Heart Association.)

## TREATMENT

The treatment for VF and pulseless VT is the same. Because both dysrhythmias are rapidly fatal, therapy must be instituted without delay. *Always check the patient before intervening, because the artifact created by loose leads can be a convincing mimic of VF.*

1. Administer a precordial thump (witnessed arrest in a monitored patient only).
2. If a defibrillator is immediately available, defibrillate starting at 200 joules of delivered energy; if unsuccessful, the energy for subsequent shocks should be increased to 300 joules and finally to 360 joules.

   **Note:** If a defibrillator is not immediately available, institute CPR without delay.

3. Begin cardiopulmonary resuscitation (CPR).
4. Establish an airway and oxygenate (which may require emergent intubation).
5. Establish venous access.
6. Administer drugs including epinephrine, xylocaine, procainamide, bretylium, and magnesium.

   **Note:** Bretylium is sometimes called a chemical defibrillator because it can facilitate defibrillation in the absence of electrical shock.

7. Continue CPR, attempt to defibrillate again every few minutes, and continue drug therapy.

---

### BOX 9–4  Signal-Averaged ECG

A signal-averaged ECG is a noninvasive test used to predict those patients who are at risk for developing VT and sudden cardiac death. Candidates for signal averaging include those with a history of myocardial infarction, cardiomyopathy, and unexplained syncope.

Signal averaging is designed to expose signals called late potentials (LPs) that are generated at reentry sites within the heart. Reentry is the mechanism most often implicated in VT. Signals recorded from reentry sites are not visible on the conventional 12-lead ECG because they are extremely small. The signal-averaged ECG analyzes multiple QRS complexes and reveals magnified LPs by eliminating extraneous signals ("noise" produced by muscle, electronics, and so on).

The patient is supine and quiet to minimize muscle artifact during the test. The skin is prepared, and surface ECG electrodes are applied in orthogonal positions (X, Y, Z). At least 200 QRS complexes are computer averaged, and the result is evaluated for the presence of LPs. Three parameters are assessed:

BOX 9-4 (continued)

1. **Total QRS duration** (greater than 110 msec is abnormal).
2. **Duration of the portion of terminal QRS with amplitude less than 40 mV** (greater than 40 msec is abnormal).
3. **Root mean square of the terminal 40 msec** (less than 20 $\mu$V is abnormal).

Note that the prognostic value of the signal-averaged ECG is altered in the presence of bundle branch block, nonspecific intraventricular conduction delay, paced rhythms, and selected antidysrhythmic drugs.

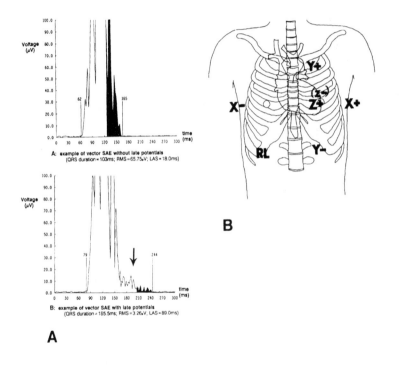

Signal-averaged ECG. (A) Note the late potentials exposed in the bottom sample (*arrow*). (B) Orthogonal lead placement for a signal-averaged ECG. (From Moser, DK, Woo, MA, and Stevenson, WG: Noninvasive identification of patients at risk for ventricular tachycardia with the signal averaged electrocardiogram. Clinical Issues in Critical Care Nursing 1:80, 1990, with permission.)

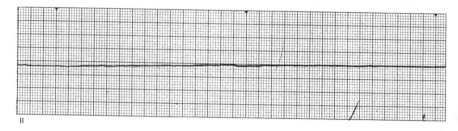

**FIGURE 9-15.** Ventricular asystole. There are no identifiable waveforms, and the baseline appears flat. Asystole cannot be differentiated from VF in the absence of ECG monitoring. (From Brown, KR and Jacobson, S: Mastering Dysrhythmias: A Problem-Solving Guide. FA Davis, Philadelphia, 1988, p 129, with permission.)

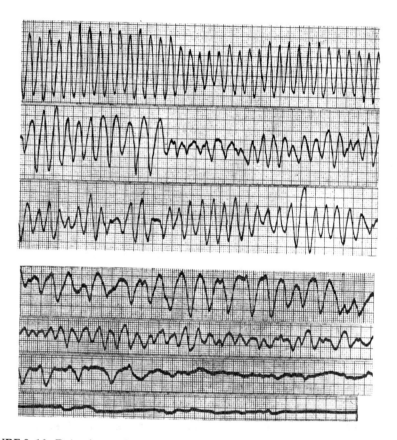

**FIGURE 9-16.** Dying heart. Continuous strip of lead II. Note onset in top lead of episode of ventricular flutter with regular oscillatory waves (no isoelectric baseline or T waves identified) changing to irregular undulating waves characteristic of ventricular fibrillation, ending with a straight line. Old tracing was taken before the era of defibrillators. Note episode of Torsade de pointes in center of second strip. (From Dunn, MI and Lipman, BS: Lipman-Massie Clinical Electrocardiography. Year Book Medical Publishers, Chicago, 1989, p 434, with permission.)

# ❒ VENTRICULAR ASYSTOLE

## DEFINITION

Ventricular asystole is characterized by the complete absence of electrical activity in the heart. Asystole (also called cardiac standstill) represents the terminal cardiac event in a variety of disease states. Without ECG monitoring, it cannot be distinguished from VF.

## ETIOLOGY

1. Failure of normal intrinsic cardiac pacemakers (owing to drugs, acute myocardial infarction, and so forth)
2. Protracted episode of VF

## CHARACTERISTICS

1. No ECG waveforms are identifiable.
2. Baseline appears flat. Because asystole may be confused with fine VF, confirm asystole by examining a different lead.

## TREATMENT

1. Institute CPR without delay.
2. Administer IV epinephrine or atropine.
3. Initiate external (transcutaneous) pacing as soon as possible.

   **Note:** Do not shock the patient in ventricular asystole.

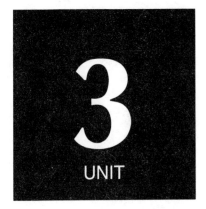

# HEART BLOCKS

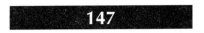

**Heart blocks** represent conduction disturbances that originate in the sinus node, the atrioventricular (AV) node, or the bundle branch system. Symptoms associated with heart block are usually a reflection of their impact on the overall ventricular rate.

# Chapter

# 10

# SINOATRIAL BLOCK

## ❏ DEFINITION

Sinoatrial (SA) block represents impaired conduction from the SA node to the atria. This results in no depolarization of the atria and absence of the entire P-QRS-T complex.

## ❏ ETIOLOGY

1. Increased vagal tone
2. Inferior wall myocardial infarction
3. Age-related degeneration of the electrical conduction system (senile degeneration)
4. Drugs such as digoxin, beta blockers, calcium blockers, and class IA antidysrhythmic agents
5. Hyperkalemia
6. Myocarditis

## ❏ CHARACTERISTICS

1. The R-R interval is irregular because an entire P-QRS-T complex is dropped, creating a pause on the ECG. Spread of the sinus impulse to the atria is blocked, so that the atria (and subsequently the ventricles as well) are never depolarized.
2. The P-P interval surrounding the pause is commonly a multiple of the previous P-P intervals.
3. If more than one sinus cycle is dropped, the pause between complexes can be lengthy. If the pause is long enough, atrial, junctional, or ventricular escape beats may be observed.

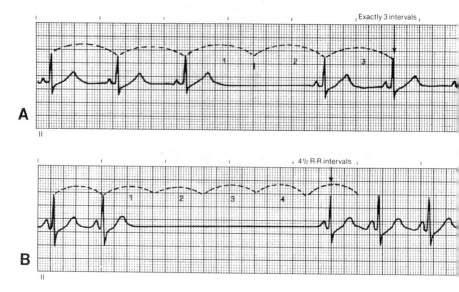

**FIGURE 10-1.** SA block and sinus arrest. (*A*) SA block. The sinus impulse fails to depolarize the atria, so an entire P-QRS-T complex is dropped. The P-P (and R-R) interval surrounding the pause is a multiple of the underlying P-P (and R-R) interval. (*B*) Sinus arrest. The sinus impulse fails to discharge, resulting in a pause that is **not** a multiple of the underlying P-P (and R-R) interval. (From Brown, KR and Jacobson, S: Mastering Dysrhythmias: A Problem-Solving Guide. FA Davis, Philadelphia, 1988, p 42, with permission.)

SA block is different from **sinus arrest.** The latter implies complete failure of the sinus node to discharge an impulse. Sinus arrest also results in loss of an entire P-QRS-T complex, but the duration of the pause is variable.

## ☐ TREATMENT

1. Determine the cause.
2. Administer atropine (if necessary).
3. Insert a pacemaker (if indicated).

**CLINICAL TIP**
SA block or sinus arrest may be an early manifestation of **sick sinus syndrome,** a condition characterized by alternating periods of bradycardia and tachycardia, sinus arrest, and failure of escape pacemakers. Sick sinus syndrome is often manifested by symptoms of weakness, dizziness, and presyncope.

# Chapter

# 11

# ATRIOVENTRICULAR BLOCKS

Atrioventricular (AV) blocks represent prolonged, intermittent, or absent conduction between the atria and the ventricles.

## ❐ FIRST-DEGREE AV BLOCK

### DEFINITION

First-degree AV block represents consistently prolonged conduction between the atria and the ventricles. It is characterized by a partial block within the AV node resulting in prolongation of the PR interval and preservation of the underlying rhythm.

### ETIOLOGY

1. Drugs (digoxin, beta blockers, calcium channel blockers, class IC antidysrhythmic agents)
2. Increased vagal tone
3. Hyperkalemia
4. Myocardial infarction (especially inferior wall myocardial infarction)
5. Myocarditis
6. Degeneration of conducting pathways associated with aging
7. Idiopathic causes

### CHARACTERISTICS

1. The PR interval is greater than 0.20 second in an adult.
2. The length of the prolonged PR interval is constant.
3. Each P wave is followed by a QRS complex (intact AV conduction).

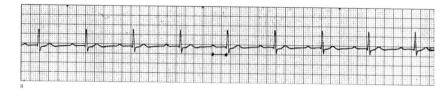

**FIGURE 11-1.** First-degree AV block. The PR interval is consistently prolonged at 0.32 second. The underlying rhythm is sinus bradycardia. (From Brown, KR and Jacobson, S: Mastering Dysrhythmias: A Problem-Solving Guide. FA Davis, Philadelphia, 1988, p 223, with permission.)

## TREATMENT

Because first-degree AV block is usually not associated with untoward symptoms, specific treatment is usually not indicated.

### ⬜ CLINICAL TIP

The lengthening of the PR interval should be evaluated over time. Because prolongation of the PR interval can occur with drugs such as digitalis, the appearance of first-degree AV block is no cause for alarm. However, if the PR interval lengthens drastically, the possibility of drug toxicity should be investigated.

# ☐ SECOND-DEGREE AV BLOCK, TYPE I

## DEFINITION

Second-degree AV block type I (also known as **Mobitz type I** or **Wenckebach**) reflects intermittent conduction between the atria and the ventricles. The location of the block is found most often within the AV node. Usually a transient disturbance, type I second-degree AV block rarely produces untoward symptoms.

## ETIOLOGY

1. Digitalis
2. Excessive vagal tone
3. Inferior wall myocardial infarction
4. Ischemic heart disease
5. Myocarditis
6. Normal variant (especially in athletes)

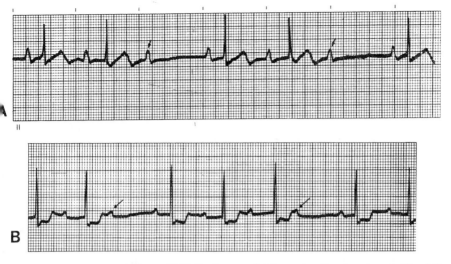

**FIGURE 11-2.** Second-degree AV block, type I. Group beating is present. The PR intervals lengthen until a beat is dropped *(arrows)*. The QRS complexes are narrow. *(A)* The nonconducted P waves *(arrows)* are easily visible. (From Brown, KR and Jacobson, S: Mastering Dysrhythmias: A Problem-Solving Guide. FA Davis, Philadelphia, 1988, p 18, with permission.) *(B)* The nonconducted P wave distorts the T wave of the preceding QRS complex. (Reproduced with permission. Textbook of Advanced Cardiac Life Support, p 81, 1987. Copyright American Heart Association.)

## CHARACTERISTICS

1. *Progressive lengthening of the PR interval until a QRS complex is dropped;* the P wave appears on time, but no QRS follows.
2. The first PR interval in a group of beats may be normal or prolonged. Subsequent PR intervals lengthen in smaller and smaller increments. *As the PR intervals get longer, the R-R intervals get shorter.*
3. P-P intervals are constant.
4. The R-R interval is irregular owing to the dropped beats, causing the QRS complexes to appear clustered together. This phenomenon, called **grouped beating,** is a hallmark of type I second-degree AV block.
5. The QRS complex is narrow unless intraventricular conduction is disturbed.
6. The conduction ratio (P to QRS) may vary. AV conduction is most often 1:1 with dropped QRS complexes appearing intermittently. However, AV conduction may be 2:1 (two P waves for every QRS complex), 3:1, or greater.

## TREATMENT

Because most patients remain asymptomatic, definitive therapy is usually unnecessary.

1. If drug toxicity is the cause, withhold the offending drug.
2. An artificial pacemaker can be used as an electrical backup if worsening heart block is expected.
3. If rate-related symptoms appear (e.g., weakness, lightheadedness, or syncope), the underlying sinus rate can be cautiously accelerated through administration of atropine.

# □ SECOND-DEGREE AV BLOCK, TYPE II

## DEFINITION

Second-degree AV block type II (also known as **Mobitz type II**) reflects intermittent and sudden loss of conduction between the atria and the ventricles. The location of the block is found most often **below** the bundle of His (within the bundle branch system). Type II second-degree AV block is a potentially dangerous condition that can progress to complete heart block (see p 156) or ventricular asystole without warning.

## ETIOLOGY

1. Acute myocardial infarction (especially anterior wall myocardial infarction)
2. Drugs (e.g., digitalis, beta blockers, calcium blockers)
3. Degeneration of the electrical conduction system (sick sinus syndrome), which is usually age-related

## CHARACTERISTICS

1. The PR interval remains constant, or fixed. Although the PR interval may be normal or prolonged, it does not vary because the basic cause of type II block is *below* the AV node.
2. The P-P interval remains regular.
3. The R-R interval is irregular because of the intermittent and sudden appearance of dropped beats. The P wave appears on time, but no QRS follows.
4. The QRS complex is usually wider than normal because of associated conduction block in the ventricles (intraventricular conduction delay [IVCD]).
5. The conduction ratio may vary. Atrioventricular conduction is often 1:1 with only intermittent dropped QRS complexes. However, rela-

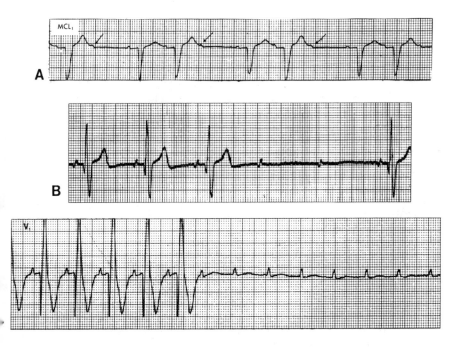

**FIGURE 11-3.** Second-degree AV block, type II. The PR intervals remain fixed. The QRS complexes are wider than normal. (*A*) The nonconducted P waves are visible in the terminal portion of the T wave. (From Marriott, HJL and Conover, MB: Advanced Concepts in Arrhythmias, ed 2. CV Mosby, St. Louis, 1989, p 249, with permission.) (*B*) The ventricular rate slows to 20 bpm when all conduction pathways into the ventricles are blocked. Conduction resumes after a pause of just over 3 seconds. (Reproduced with permission. Textbook of Advanced Cardiac Life Support, 1987, p 82. Copyright American Heart Association.) (*C*) The wide QRS complex indicates a preexisting conduction disturbance in the bundle branches. Complete block of the conduction pathways into the ventricles results in ventricular asystole (with no escape pacemaker). (Reproduced with permission. Textbook of Advanced Cardiac Life Support, 1987, p 84. Copyright American Heart Association.)

tively fixed conduction ratios such as 2:1 (two P waves for every QRS complex), 3:1, or greater may be seen.

## TREATMENT

Because second-degree AV block type II may be very serious, treatment depends on the clinical situation.

1. Withhold possible causative drugs.
2. Atropine can be given to accelerate the underlying sinus rate if rate-related symptoms appear.

3. Temporary or permanent pacemaker insertion is often performed because type II block may deteriorate suddenly to third-degree AV block.

🗒 **CLINICAL TIP**

Rate is much more important than ratio when describing AV blocks with fixed conduction ratios such as 2:1, 3:1, or more. For example, 2:1 AV block implies two P waves for every QRS, but the description is incomplete for it fails to address rate. If the underlying sinus rate is 200, the ventricular response is a tolerable 100. On the other hand, a sinus rate of 70 results in a ventricular rate of 35, which may be a clinical emergency. The "2:1 AV block" label, without its rate qualifier, is insufficient.

# ◻ THIRD-DEGREE AV BLOCK

## DEFINITION

Third-degree AV block (also known as **complete heart block** [CHB]) represents complete absence of conduction between atria and ventricles. An **escape** pacemaker below the level of the block may take over at a slower rate. CHB is characterized by independent beating between atria and ventricles (this is an example of AV dissociation; see p 158). In other words, P waves appear at one rate, whereas QRS complexes, unrelated to the P waves, appear at a slower rate.

## ETIOLOGY

1. Drug toxicity (e.g., digoxin, beta blockers, calcium blockers)
2. Excessive vagal tone
3. Acute myocardial infarction
4. Age-related degeneration of the electrical conduction system
5. Myocarditis
6. Endocarditis
7. Cardiac surgery
8. Congenital origin

## CHARACTERISTICS

1. P-P intervals are usually constant.
2. R-R intervals are usually constant.
3. The atrial and ventricular rates are different (the atrial rate is usually faster than the ventricular rate).
4. There is no relationship between the P waves and the QRS complexes. Because the P waves "march through" the QRS complexes, some P

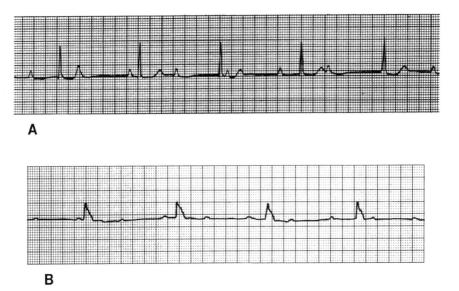

**A**

**B**

**FIGURE 11-4.** Third-degree AV block. The P-P and R-R intervals are nearly regular, but the atrial and ventricular rates are different. There is no relationship between the P waves and the QRS complexes. (*A*) Third-degree AV block with a junctional escape pacemaker. The QRS complexes are narrow, and the ventricular rate is 44 bpm. (*B*) Third-degree AV block with a ventricular escape pacemaker. The QRS complexes are wide, and the ventricular rate is 37 bpm. (Reproduced with permission. Textbook of Advanced Cardiac Life Support, 1987, p 83. Copyright American Heart Association.)

waves will be hidden within QRS complexes and others may deform them.

5. Both the width of the QRS complex and the ventricular rate reflect the location of the escape pacemaker. If CHB exists at the level of the AV node, a junctional escape pacemaker will normally fire at 40 to 60 bpm, and the QRS complex will be narrow (assuming normal intraventricular conduction). If CHB exists within the bundle branch system, a ventricular escape pacemaker will fire at 15 to 40 bpm, and the QRS complex will be wide.

## TREATMENT

Because third-degree AV block is often accompanied by rate-related symptoms, therapy is designed either to accelerate conduction through the AV node or to support the ventricular rate.

1. Administer atropine in an attempt to restore conduction through the AV node.
2. Administer epinephrine for short-term rate support.

3. If the block is due to drug toxicity, withhold the offending drug.
4. Insert a pacemaker. Temporary pacing is most appropriate with transient block or in emergent situations. Permanent pacing may also be recommended depending on the clinical situation.

---

BOX 11-1 **Differentiating AV Blocks**

_____

AV blocks can be diagnosed without a lot of fuss and bother if you follow the guidelines described here. There are three ECG parameters to examine.

1. **Look at the R-R interval.** Is it regular or irregular?
2. **Look at the P waves.** Is there one (or more than one) P wave for every QRS complex?
3. **Look at the PR interval.** Does it stay the same or does it change?

*If the R-R interval is REGULAR, the block is probably either first degree or third degree.*

- If there is *only one P wave* for every QRS complex, if the PR intervals stay the same: **first-degree AV block**
- If there is *more than one P wave* for every QRS complex, if the PR intervals change: **third-degree AV block**

*If the R-R interval is IRREGULAR, the block is probably second degree, type I or type II.*

- If the PR intervals *change:* **second-degree AV block, type I**
- If the PR intervals *stay the same:* **second-degree AV block, type II**

**Note:** Second-degree AV block associated with multiple dropped beats can exhibit either fixed or variable conduction ratios, so the regularity of the R-R interval is not the most critical clue.

- If there is more than one P wave for every QRS, if the PR intervals stay the same: **second-degree AV block with either fixed or variable conduction** (e.g., 2:1 AV block)

BOX 11-2 **AV Dissociation**

AV dissociation is *not* a rhythm. It is a *descriptive term* characterizing any rhythm in which the atria and ventricles are dissociated, or controlled by completely separate pacemakers.
There are several situations in which AV dissociation is found:

1. **When the sinus rate is slower than the escape rate of a subsidiary pacemaker.** An example is sinus bradycardia (rate of 40 bpm) with a junctional pacemaker (rate of 55 bpm). The atria are driven by the sinus pacemaker and the ventricles by the junctional pacemaker.

2. **When the sinus rate is slower than the rate of an enhanced subsidiary pacemaker.** An example is sinus rhythm (rate of 60 bpm) with an accelerated junctional (rate of 70 bpm) or ventricular pacemaker (rate of 65 bpm). The enhanced subsidiary pacemaker overrides the sinus pacemaker.

3. **When third-degree (complete) AV block exists.** The atria are driven by the sinus pacemaker (rate of 80 bpm) and the ventricles by either a junctional or a ventricular pacemaker (rate of 40 bpm). An example is sinus rhythm with complete heart block and a ventricular escape pacemaker.

# 12

# BUNDLE BRANCH BLOCKS

Bundle branch blocks represent defects in **intraventricular** conduction that usually produce no untoward symptoms. The supraventricular impulse emerging from the bundle of His proceeds down the unblocked bundle branch and depolarizes one ventricle. On the side of the bundle branch block, the impulse spreads slowly through the ventricular muscle resulting in abnormal depolarization. The abnormally wide QRS complex that results is the hallmark of bundle branch block.

## ☐ RIGHT BUNDLE BRANCH BLOCK

### DEFINITION

Right bundle branch block (RBBB) results from a conduction delay or block within the right bundle branch.

### ETIOLOGY

1. Right ventricular hypertrophy
2. Right ventricular strain (due to acute pulmonary embolism, acute or chronic lung disease).
3. Atrial septal defect
4. Wolff-Parkinson-White (WPW) syndrome, type A (causes a pseudo-RBBB pattern; see p 233).
5. Coronary artery disease
6. Myocarditis
7. Cardiac contusion
8. Idiopathic causes

I    II    III    aVR    aVL    aVF

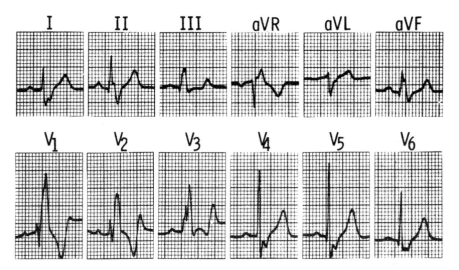

V₁    V₂    V₃    V₄    V₅    V₆

**FIGURE 12-1.** Right bundle branch block. The QRS complex is wide and predominantly positive in lead $V_1$. Note the classic rsR′ configuration of the QRS in right-sided chest leads $V_1$ and $V_2$. The onset of the intrinsicoid deflection is also delayed in the right chest leads. A wide S wave is visible in left-sided leads I, aVL, $V_5$, and $V_6$. (From Chung, EK and Chung, DK: ECG Diagnosis: Self-Assessment. Harper & Row, Hagerstown, MD, 1972, with permission.

## CHARACTERISTICS

1. The QRS complex is 0.12 second or more in width.

   **Note:** If the QRS duration is equal to or greater than 0.12 second, the block is called complete RBBB, but if it falls between 0.10 and 0.12 second, the block is called incomplete RBBB.

2. The QRS complex is predominantly positive and often assumes an rsR′ (or "rabbit ear") morphology in right precordial leads $V_1$ and $V_2$. The initial r wave represents normal left-to-right septal depolarization; the S wave represents depolarization of the left ventricle ($V_1$ records a negative deflection because it "sees" the depolarization current moving *away from* its positive end); the R′ ("R prime") wave represents delayed activation of the right ventricle ($V_1$ records a second positive deflection because it "sees" the depolarization current moving *toward* its positive end).

3. A wide or deep S wave in left-sided leads I, aVL, $V_5$, and $V_6$ represents delayed activation of the right ventricle.

4. A downsloping ST segment and inverted T wave in leads $V_1$ and $V_2$ represent secondary repolarization changes.

5. The time of onset of the intrinsicoid deflection* (measured from the beginning of the QRS complex to the peak of the R wave) is delayed in the right ventricular leads but is normal in the left ventricular leads.

## 🔲 CLINICAL TIP

Leads representing the ventricle with the conduction block will record a delayed onset of the intrinsicoid deflection, whereas leads representing the normal ventricle will record a normal onset of the intrinsicoid deflection. The normal onset of the intrinsicoid deflection in the left-sided leads (I, aVL, $V_5$, and $V_6$) is approximately 0.04 second; it is approximately 0.02 second in the right-sided leads ($V_1$ and $V_2$).

## TREATMENT

There is no treatment for RBBB.

# ☐ LEFT BUNDLE BRANCH BLOCK

## DEFINITION

Left bundle branch block (LBBB) results from a conduction delay or block within the left bundle branch.

## ETIOLOGY

1. Left ventricular hypertrophy
2. Cardiomyopathy
3. Hypertension
4. Coronary artery disease
5. Myocarditis
6. WPW syndrome, type B (causes a pseudo-LBBB pattern; see p 233).

## CHARACTERISTICS

1. The QRS complex is 0.12 second or more in width.

    **Note:** If the QRS duration is equal to or greater than 0.12 second, the block is called complete LBBB, but if it falls between 0.10 and 0.12 second, the block is called incomplete LBBB.

2. The QRS complex is predominantly negative in right chest leads $V_1$ and $V_2$. A wide, deep S wave makes up the majority of the QRS complex and represents delayed activation of the left ventricle.

---

*The intrinsicoid deflection is the initial downward deflection after the peak of the R wave.

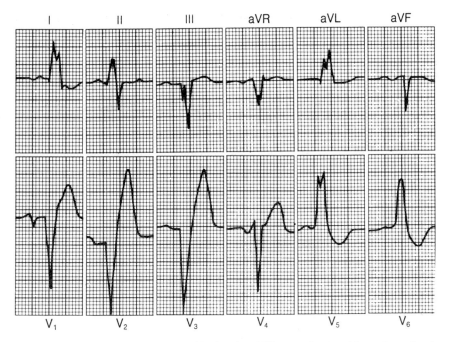

**FIGURE 12–2.** Left bundle branch block. The QRS complex is wide and predominantly negative in lead $V_1$. The QRS complex in the left-sided leads assumes a rabbit-ear shape. The onset of the intrinsicoid deflection is also delayed in the left chest leads. (From Wilson, RF: Critical Care Manual: Applied Physiology and Principles of Therapy, ed 2. FA Davis, Philadelphia, 1992, p 157, with permission.)

3. The QRS complex often assumes a positive rsR′ (or "rabbit ear") morphology in leads I, aVL, $V_5$, and $V_6$. The initial r wave represents abnormal right-to-left septal depolarization; the s wave represents right ventricular depolarization; and the R′ deflection represents delayed activation of the left ventricle.

4. The ST segment and T wave are oriented in the opposite direction to the main QRS. They are called secondary ST-T changes and are normally found in LBBB. These changes are often mistaken for myocardial ischemia or injury.

5. The time of onset of the intrinsicoid deflection is delayed in the left ventricular leads (I, aVL, $V_5$, and $V_6$), but it is normal in the right ventricular leads.

## TREATMENT

Treatment of LBBB is usually unnecessary. However, in the setting of an acute event (such as myocardial infarction), other rhythm disturbances such as atrioventricular block may develop that would require specific intervention.

☐ **CLINICAL TIP**
The most useful leads for diagnosis of bundle branch blocks are $V_1$ and $V_6$.

---

BOX 12-1 **Differentiating Bundle Branch Blocks**

**RBBB**
- QRS wide and predominantly positive in lead $V_1$
- rSR' in lead $V_1$ (rabbit ears)
- Deep S in lead $V_6$ (and lead I)
- Late intrinsicoid deflection in lead $V_1$, normal in lead $V_6$

**LBBB**
- QRS wide and predominantly negative in lead $V_1$
- rSR' in lead $V_6$ (and lead I)
- rS or QS in lead $V_1$
- Late intrinsicoid deflection in lead $V_6$, normal in lead $V_1$

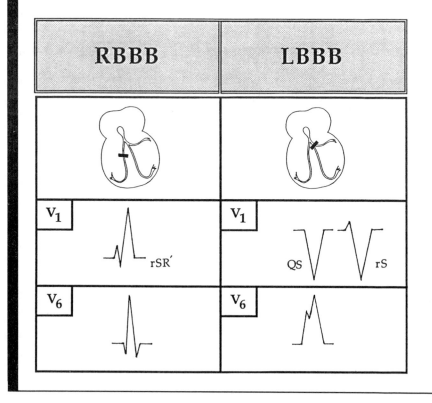

# Chapter

# 13

# FASCICULAR BLOCKS

Fascicular blocks (also known as hemiblocks) represent disturbed conduction in either the anterior or the posterior division, or fascicle, of the left bundle branch.

## ☐ LEFT ANTERIOR FASCICULAR BLOCK

### DEFINITION

Left anterior fascicular block (LAFB), also called left anterior hemiblock, represents a delay in conduction through the anterior fascicle of the left bundle branch. LAFB is more common than left posterior fascicular block (LPFB). The anterior fascicle is long and thin and has a single blood supply, which makes it more vulnerable to block than the posterior fascicle.

### ETIOLOGY

1. Coronary artery disease
2. Myocardial infarction
3. Congenital heart disease
4. Cardiac surgery
5. Aging process
6. Normal variant

### CHARACTERISTICS

1. The duration of the QRS may be slightly prolonged (between 0.08 and 0.11 second).

| I | II | III | aVR | aVL | aVF |

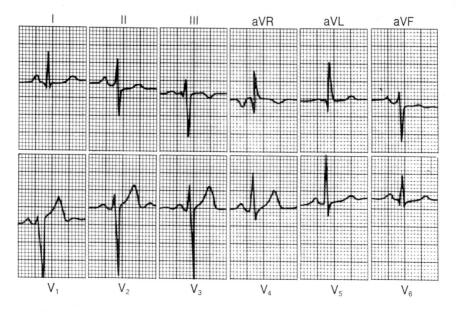

| $V_1$ | $V_2$ | $V_3$ | $V_4$ | $V_5$ | $V_6$ |

**FIGURE 13–1.** Left anterior fascicular block. There is a small q and tall R in leads I and aVL. A small r and deep S are visible in leads II, III, and aVF. Left axis deviation is present. (From Wilson, RF: Critical Care Manual: Applied Physiology and Principles of Therapy, ed 2. FA Davis, Philadelphia, 1992, p 159, with permission.)

2. Left axis deviation (LAD) is present; the QRS axis ranges between −45° and −90°. LAD is caused by the late, abnormal depolarization of the portion of the left ventricle normally depolarized by the left anterior fascicle.

3. A small q wave and a tall R wave are visible in leads I and aVL. The small q wave represents conduction down the unblocked posterior fascicle; the tall R wave represents delayed depolarization of the anterior portion of the left ventricle as the impulse spreads through the muscle.

4. A small r wave and a deep S wave are visible in leads II, III, and aVF. The small r wave represents initial conduction down the posterior fascicle, and the deep S wave represents delayed depolarization of the anterior left ventricle.

5. Poor R-wave progression in the precordial leads.

🔋 **CLINICAL TIP**

Because the hallmark of LAFB is LAD, other causes of LAD (e.g., inferior wall myocardial infarction, obstructive lung disease, hypertrophic cardiomyopathy, and Wolff-Parkinson-White [WPW] syndrome) should be excluded before the label "LAFB" is applied.

## TREATMENT

Treatment is not indicated. However, evaluation of the underlying cause may be important, especially in the acute setting.

## ◻ LEFT POSTERIOR FASCICULAR BLOCK

### DEFINITION

Left posterior fascicular block (LPFB), also called left posterior hemiblock, represents a delay in conduction through the posterior division of the left bundle branch. The posterior fascicle is short, thick, and enjoys a double blood supply, making it less susceptible to injury than the anterior fascicle. The appearance of LPFB usually implies that a large amount of myocardial injury has occurred, so the implications of LPFB are more serious than with LAFB.

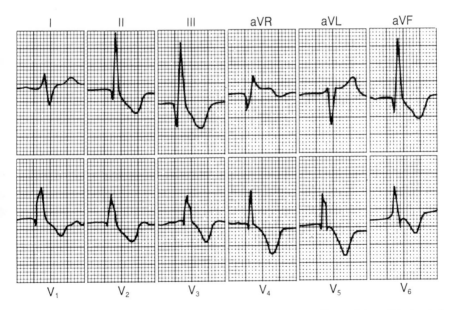

**FIGURE 13–2.** Left posterior fascicular block. There is a small r and deep S in leads I and aVL. A small q and tall R are visible in leads II, III, and aVF. Right axis deviation is present. In this tracing, right bundle branch block is also present. (From Wilson, RF: Critical Care Manual: Applied Physiology and Principles of Therapy, ed 2. FA Davis, Philadelphia, 1992, p 159, with permission.)

## ETIOLOGY

1. Coronary artery disease
2. Myocardial infarction
3. Congenital heart disease
4. Cardiac surgery

## CHARACTERISTICS

1. The duration of the QRS complex is slightly prolonged (between 0.08 and 0.11 second).
2. Right axis deviation (RAD) is present; the QRS axis ranges between +90° and +180°. RAD is caused by the late, abnormal depolarization of the portion of the left ventricle normally depolarized by the left posterior fascicle.
3. A small q wave and a tall R wave are visible in leads II, III, and aVF. The small q wave represents conduction down the unblocked anterior fascicle; the tall R wave represents delayed depolarization of the posterior portion of the left ventricle as the impulse spreads through the muscle.
4. A small r wave and a deep S wave are visible in leads I and aVL. The small r wave represents initial conduction down the anterior fascicle, and the deep S wave represents delayed depolarization of the posterior left ventricle.

### CLINICAL TIP
Because the hallmark of LPFB is RAD, other causes of RAD (e.g., lateral wall myocardial infarction, obstructive lung disease) should be excluded before the label "LPFB" is applied.

## TREATMENT

Treatment is usually unnecessary; however, the appearance of LPFB during a myocardial infarction implies extensive muscle damage that may lead to significant dysrhythmias and heart failure.

### CLINICAL TIP
The best leads for evaluating fascicular blocks are limb leads because they reveal important axis shifts.

BOX 13-1 **Differentiating Fascicular Blocks**

**LAFB**
- LAD
- qR in lead I
- rS in lead III

**LPFB**
- RAD
- qR in lead III
- rS in lead I

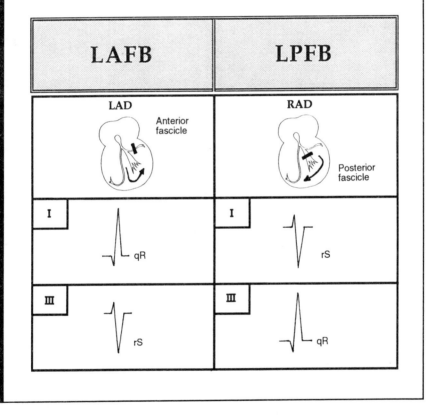

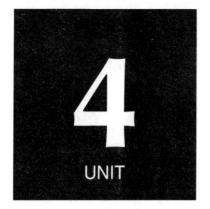

**UNIT**

# ARTIFICIAL PACEMAKERS

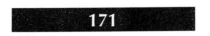

# Chapter

# 14

# ARTIFICIAL PACEMAKERS

An artificial pacemaker is an electronic device that creates and transmits an electrical signal to the atria, the ventricles, or both. Most artificial pacemakers function like electrical backup systems that keep the heart rate fast enough to prevent rate-related clinical symptoms. Pacemakers may be implanted on a temporary or permanent basis, depending on the clinical situation. More complex devices are incorporated with antitachycardia and defibrillator features designed to abolish rapid dysrhythmias.

## ☐ INDICATIONS FOR CONVENTIONAL PACING

### TEMPORARY PACING

Temporary pacing is appropriate in emergent situations (e.g., ventricular asystole) or if there is a risk of symptomatic bradycardia, as in patients with transient atrioventricular (AV) block (associated with cardiac surgery, myocardial ischemia, or drug toxicity).

### PERMANENT PACING

Permanent pacemaker implantation does not automatically follow temporary pacing. The procedure is warranted only after careful analysis of each patient's clinical situation. Permanent pacing is considered in the following circumstances:*

1. Acquired AV block
   a. Acquired complete AV block

---

*Adapted from American College of Cardiology/American Heart Association Task Force: Guidelines for implantation of cardiac pacemakers and antiarrhythmia devices: A report of the American College of Cardiology/American Heart Association task force on assessment of diagnostic and therapeutic cardiovascular procedures (committee on pacemaker implantation). J Am Coll Cardiol 18(1):1, 1991.

**b.** Second-degree AV block accompanied by symptomatic bradycardia

**c.** Atrial fibrillation or atrial flutter associated with advanced or complete heart block (unrelated to drugs known to impair AV conduction)

2. AV block associated with myocardial infarction

**a.** Persistent advanced second-degree AV block or complete heart block with block in the His-Purkinje system (bilateral bundle branch block) following acute myocardial infarction

**b.** Transient advanced AV block with associated bundle branch block

3. Chronic bifascicular or trifascicular block

**a.** Bifascicular block with intermittent complete heart block and symptomatic bradycardia

**b.** Bifascicular or trifascicular block with intermittent type II second-degree AV block (symptoms not necessary)

4. Sick sinus syndrome: Sinus node dysfunction (sinus bradycardia, sinus arrest, sinoatrial [SA] block) accompanied by clinical symptoms (e.g., dizziness or syncope)

5. Hypersensitive carotid sinus: Recurrent syncope provoked by carotid sinus stimulation (asystole longer than 3 seconds in the absence of drugs that depress sinus node or AV conduction)

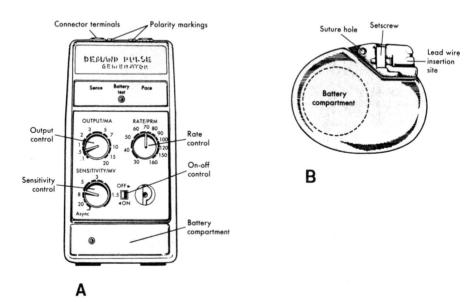

**FIGURE 14–1.** Examples of pulse generators. (*A*) Temporary generator. Controls on the face of the unit allow operator manipulation of pacing parameters. Removable batteries are contained within the generator housing. (*B*) Permanent generator. Pacing parameters are set during the implantation procedure or by a programmer placed directly over the generator. (From Beare, PG and Myers, JL: Principles and Practice of Adult Health Nursing. CV Mosby, St. Louis, 1990, p 793, with permission.)

# ☐ COMPONENTS

All pacemakers share common components, the pulse generator and the pacing catheter.

- The **pulse generator** contains batteries that create the electrical signal. Most permanent generators are driven by lithium batteries that last from 2 to 10 years before a replacement is needed. Temporary generators run on removable batteries that are changed periodically.
- The **pacing catheter** (often called the lead or the electrode) is the link between the source of the electrical signal (the pulse generator) and the myocardium. It is a **two-way** transmission line that delivers the electrical stimulus to the heart and conducts information about intrinsic electrical activity back to the generator for processing. Many permanent pacing catheters are constructed with fixation devices (e.g., screws, tines, or barbs) that help guarantee long-term contact with the wall of the heart. Temporary catheters are constructed for easy removal when pacing is no longer required.

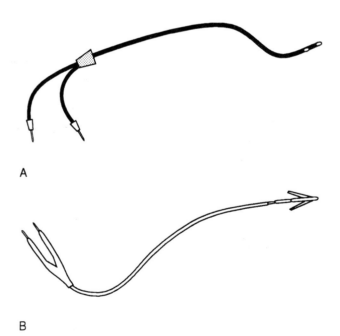

A

B

**FIGURE 14–2.** Examples of pacing catheters. (*A*) Temporary catheter with no fixation device at the tip. (*B*) Permanent catheter with a fixation device (a tine in this example) on the tip of the catheter.

# ☐ INSERTION

## TEMPORARY PACING

Temporary pulse generators are externally controlled by manipulating dials on the face of the unit. The pacing catheter is commonly inserted into a vein (the transvenous approach) and is advanced until the right atrial or ventricular endocardium is reached; ideally, this is done under fluoroscopy. The catheter is connected to the external generator, pacing parameters are set, and the unit is turned on.

- In emergency situations, **transthoracic** pacing can be achieved quickly. A special pacing catheter is threaded into the ventricle through a large-bore needle that has been inserted directly into the heart through the anterior chest wall.

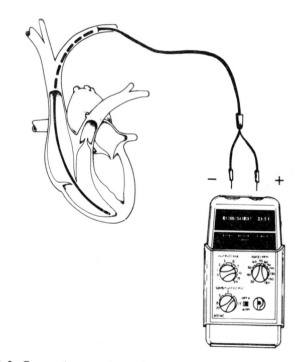

**FIGURE 14–3.** Connecting a pacing catheter to a temporary generator. The two external pins on the proximal end of a temporary pacing catheter are inserted into terminals found on the pacemaker generator. The pin marked "negative" (or distal) is inserted into the generator's negative terminal; the pin marked "positive" (or proximal) is inserted into the positive terminal. A bridging cable, or pacemaker extension cord (not shown) can be used between the generator and the catheter. (Adapted from Tucker, S, Canobbio, M, et al: Patient Care Standards, ed 5. CV Mosby, St. Louis, 1992.)

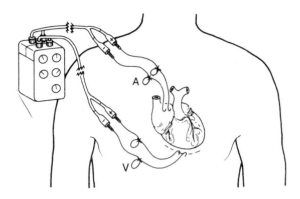

**FIGURE 14-4.** Initiating temporary pacing using surgical wires. Two to four surgical wires are normally attached to the atrium, the ventricle, or both. Atrial wires usually exit to the right of the sternum, and ventricular wires exit to the left. Pacing is initiated by inserting the wires into the appropriate terminals on a temporary pulse generator. In this example, sequential pacing (atrial pacing followed by ventricular pacing) is achieved using both atrial and ventricular wires. **Note:** If only one atrial or ventricular wire is present, insert it into the negative terminal on the pulse generator; an additional pacing wire is sutured to the outer skin surface, and the other end is inserted into the positive terminal. (From Vinsant, MO and Spence, MI: Commonsense Approach to Coronary Care: A Program, ed 5. CV Mosby, St. Louis, 1989, p 572, with permission.)

- Insulated pacing wires may be attached to the outer surface of the atrium or ventricle, or both, during cardiac surgery. These wires are externalized through the anterior chest wall. If pacing is required, the wires are attached to a temporary generator. When no longer needed, the wires are gently pulled through the wound.

## PERMANENT PACING

Permanent pulse generators are placed within a subcutaneous pocket created either in the infraclavicular area or in the abdominal wall. One end of the pacing catheter is attached to the generator, while the other end is interfaced with either the endocardial or the epicardial surface of the heart. Pacing parameters are set, the unit is turned on, and the wound is closed.

- Insertion is usually accomplished using the **transvenous** approach. The pacing catheter is inserted into a major (often the subclavian) vein and advanced into the right atrium (RA) or right ventricle (RV) until the catheter tip touches the endocardium (endocardial pacing). The procedure is associated with minimal risk, and general anesthesia is not required.
- The more complicated **transthoracic** or **transxiphisternal** surgical approach is usually reserved for situations in which conventional endocardial pacing cannot be achieved successfully. The pacing catheter is attached to the epicardial surface of the left or right ventricle

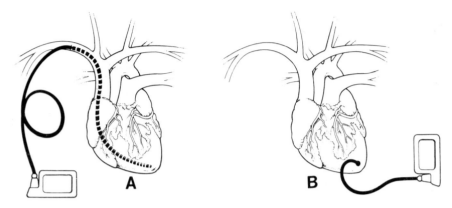

**FIGURE 14–5.** Endocardial versus epicardial pacing. (*A*) Endocardial pacing. The generator is implanted into a subcutaneous pocket in the infraclavicular area; the catheter is threaded into the right ventricle. (*B*) Epicardial pacing. The generator is implanted into a subcutaneous pocket in the abdominal wall; the catheter is affixed to the outer surface of either ventricle. (From Beare, PG and Myers, JL: Principles and Practice of Adult Health Nursing. CV Mosby, St. Louis, 1990, p 794, with permission.)

(epicardial pacing) using an abdominal approach. The operative risk is increased because general anesthesia is usually required.

**CLINICAL TIP**

Ventricular pacing causes sequential depolarization because one ventricle is stimulated before the other. If a pacing stimulus is delivered to the *left* ventricle (most commonly with epicardial or transthoracic pacing), depolarization proceeds from left ventricle to right ventricle; the resulting QRS complex resembles a right bundle branch block (RBBB) pattern (wide and predominantly positive in lead $V_1$) because depolarization of the right ventricle is delayed. If a pacing stimulus is delivered to the *right* ventricle (as in endocardial or transvenous pacing), depolarization proceeds from right to left; the resulting QRS complex resembles a left bundle branch block (LBBB) pattern (wide and predominantly negative in $V_1$) because depolarization of the left ventricle is delayed.

**Note:**   Lead $V_1$ or $MCL_1$ is recommended for continuous monitoring of the ECG in patients with pacemakers.

---

BOX 14–1 **Transcutaneous Pacing**

**Transcutaneous pacing** (also known as **external** or **transchest pacing**) refers to delivery of a pacing stimulus through electrodes applied to the chest wall. Designed for use in emergency situations (e.g., asystole or symptomatic bradycardia unresponsive to drugs), transcutaneous pacing in either the demand or the fixed-rate mode can be achieved quickly.

## BOX 14–1 (continued)

Several manufacturers currently market defibrillator/monitors incorporated with external pacing capabilities. Some models use a special pacing cassette inserted into a receptacle on the defibrillator. Still others display the pacing controls on the front of the unit alongside the defibrillation controls.

The procedure for initiating transcutaneous pacing is very simple. Large pacing pads are attached to the patient in either the anterior-posterior or anterior-anterior positions. A pacing cable runs from the pacing pads to the defibrillator/monitor. ECG leads are also attached to the patient at the conventional sites, and the ECG signal is delivered directly to the machine through a special patient cable. Pacing parameters (e.g., current output, pacing rate, and pacing mode) are set, the unit is turned on, and the ECG is observed for appropriate sensing. Current output (mA) is initially set to nominal levels. As it is slowly increased, the ECG is observed for evidence of capture (spike followed by wide QRS complex).

**Note:** Successful transcutaneous pacing requires a higher current output than conventional endocardial pacing. Delivery of this stronger current can cause both chest wall pain and skin burns (although the large size of the pacing pads minimizes the risk of burns).

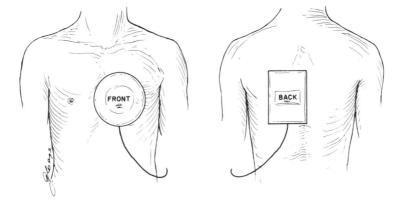

Special pacing pads are placed in either the anterior-posterior position (shown) or the anterior-anterior position on the chest wall. Excess hair is clipped before the pads are attached to maximize contact with the skin surface. The colored ends on the cable should match the color on the pacing pads (e.g., red with red, black with black). (From Clochesy, JM: Advanced Technology in Critical Care Nursing. Aspen Publishers, Rockville, MD, 1989, p 93, with permission.)

## ❑ FUNCTION

The most fundamental properties of pacemaker operation reflect the ability to sense, fire, and capture.

- **Sensing** means that the pulse generator is able to process (or "see") intrinsic electrical signals.
- **Firing** means that the pulse generator has delivered a stimulus to the heart. A pacemaker spike (or stimulus artifact) is usually visible on the ECG.
- **Capturing** means that the heart has responded to the stimulus (depolarization). A waveform (P wave or QRS complex) is visible after the spike. If the pacing catheter is in contact with the atrium, the spike will be followed by a P wave; if it is in contact with the ventricle, the spike will be followed by a wide QRS complex (the QRS is wide because the ventricles are depolarized in sequence).

The actual programming of these basic instructions involves manipulation of several key pacing parameters that are described here:

- The **automatic interval** refers to the pacing rate, or the interval between consecutive paced events. It is set either in milliseconds (msec) or in beats per minute (bpm).
- The **escape interval** (also called the demand interval) is usually the same as the automatic interval, unless **hysteresis** is present. The atrial escape interval (AEI) is the time between atrial paced events which may be reset by premature beats; the ventricular escape interval (VEI) is the time between ventricular paced events which may be reset by premature beats.
- **Hysteresis** is a feature incorporated into single chamber permanent generators that allows programming of a longer escape interval between a sensed intrinsic event and the first paced event. It is only slightly longer than the automatic interval. Hysteresis allows the artificial pacemaker to delay firing a little longer than the automatic interval in the hope that the natural sinus pacemaker will fire. If the sinus pacemaker does take over, the artificial pacemaker will not have to fire, and battery life will be preserved.
- **Milliamperes (mA)** reflect the strength of the output signal. The signal must be strong enough to cause depolarization (capture), but not so strong as to cause diaphragmatic or phrenic nerve pacing, or unnecessary depletion of the pacemaker battery.

   **Note:** The minimum amount of current required to cause a response is called "threshold" and is determined during pacemaker insertion.

- **Sensitivity** reflects the ability of the generator to process incoming cardiac signals of differing voltages; it is programmed in millivolts

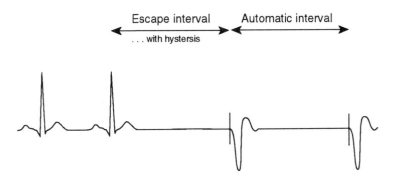

Escape interval    Automatic interval

... with hystersis

**FIGURE 14-6.** Measuring intervals. The automatic interval (also called the escape or demand interval) is measured from one paced beat to the next. In this example, hysteresis is present; the distance between the last intrinsic event and the first paced event is slightly longer than the automatic interval.

(mV). Sensitivity is easily manipulated on a temporary generator. When the sensitivity or millivolt dial is turned to the lowest number, the generator is instructed to sense virtually all intrinsic activity, even low-voltage signals. If the dial is turned to the highest number, the generator is instructed to ignore virtually all intrinsic activity, even high-voltage signals.

**Note:** The lower number on the dial correlates with demand mode pacing, whereas the higher numbers correlate with asynchronous (or fixed-rate) mode of pacing.

**CLINICAL TIP**
Over a period of days to weeks following permanent lead implantation, inflammation and fibrosis of tissue surrounding the tip of the pacing lead may raise the stimulation threshold. The milliamperes in a permanent generator are usually set higher than the initial stimulation threshold to compensate for the initial increase in threshold that accompanies lead placement. Later, the threshold usually comes back down.

# ☐ CODING

A universal five-letter coding system—a kind of pacemaker shorthand—is used to describe the function of most pacing systems. The first three letters describe fundamental operations, whereas the last two refer to more sophisticated features incorporated into some permanent generators.

1. **The first letter refers to the chamber(s) *paced*.** The pacing stimulus (or spike) will be followed by either a P wave or a QRS complex, depending on the location of the pacing catheter.

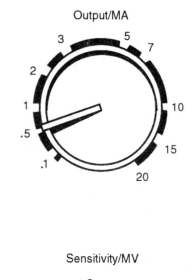

Output/MA

A

Sensitivity/MV

B

**FIGURE 14–7.** Selecting mA and sensitivity on a temporary generator. (*A*) The output/mA dial controls the strength of the output signal; turning the dial to a higher number increases the mA. (*B*) The sensitivity/mV dial controls the ability of the generator to sense intrinsic electrical activity. Turning it to a lower number increases the sensitivity. Conversely, turning it to a higher number decreases the sensitivity. The asynchronous setting allows no sensing at all.

**Note:** If both chambers are paced, the designation "D" (for double or dual) is used.

2. **The second letter refers to the chamber(s)** *sensed.* The location of the catheter determines whether intrinsic atrial or ventricular activity is sensed. For example, a catheter located in the atrium will sense atrial impulses (P waves), whereas a catheter located in the ventricle will sense ventricular impulses (including normal and ectopic QRS complexes).

**Note:** If both chambers are sensed, the designation "D" (for double or dual) is used. If sensing is absent, the designation "O" is used.

Pacemaker identification codes

| Chamber(s) paced | Chamber(s) sensed | Mode of responses (sensing function) | Programmable functions | Special tachyarrhythmia functions |
|---|---|---|---|---|
| V = Ventricle | V = Ventricle | T = Triggered | P = Programmable | B = Bursts |
| A = Atrium | A = Atrium | I = Inhibited | M = Multipro- | N = Normal rate |
| D = Double | D = Double | (demand) | grammable | competition |
| (dual) | (dual) | D = Double (dual | O = None (Perma- | (dual demand) |
| | O = None | function: T and I) | nent pacemakers | S = Scanning |
| | | O = None | only) | E = External |
| | | (continuous) | | |
| | | R = Reverse | | |

**FIGURE 14-8.** Pacemaker code. Most pacemaker functions are described using the first three letters of the code. (Adapted from Vinsant, MO and Spence, MI: Common-sense Approach to Coronary Care: A Program, ed 5. CV Mosby, St. Louis, 1989, p 575, with permission.)

3. **The third letter refers to the** *mode(s) of response.*
   - The **inhibited** mode means that the pacemaker fires "on demand." It is inhibited by intrinsic electrical signals and will not fire if these signals are sensed within a programmed escape interval. For example, a pacemaker looking for intrinsic QRS complexes will not fire if a QRS is sensed (in other words, it is inhibited by QRS complexes); however, if no QRS complex is sensed within the escape interval, the unit will fire.
   - The **triggered** mode means that the pacemaker is cued (or triggered) to fire when it senses a specific intrinsic event (a P wave or QRS complex). For example, a sensed P wave may trigger the delivery of a stimulus into the ventricle (a ventricular output).
   - The designation "D" (for double or dual) means that both the inhibited and triggered modes are operative. For a dual chamber pacemaker, this means that atrial sensing (of a P wave) *triggers* a ventricular output, and ventricular sensing (of a QRS complex) *inhibits* a ventricular output.
   - The designation "O" implies that sensing is not present. This kind of pacing, known as **asynchronous** (or fixed-rate) pacing, means that the generator fires at a preset rate, without regard to intrinsic activity.

4. **The fourth letter refers to** *programmable functions,* **or the ability to alter pacing parameters using an external device.** Pacing parameters that are commonly adjusted include the pacing rate, voltage output (mA), and sensitivity. The programmability feature of permanent pace-makers allows external adjustment of pacing parameters and spares patients the trauma of replacing pacemaker generators.

5. **The fifth letter refers to special** *antitachycardia functions.* Sophisticated antitachycardia features are designed to slow or abolish certain tachycardias.

**CLINICAL TIP**
Asynchronous (or fixed rate) pacing is rarely used in clinical prac-tice. Because a fixed rate pacemaker is programmed to ignore all

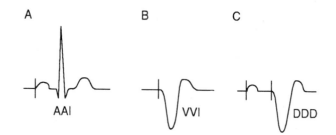

**FIGURE 14-9.** Pacemaker code examples. (*A*) AAI pacemaker. This single-chamber pacemaker looks for a P wave and fires into the atrium if no P wave is sensed; the pacing spike is followed by a P wave. (*B*) VVI pacemaker. This single-chamber pacemaker looks for a QRS complex and fires into the ventricle if no QRS is sensed; the pacing spike is followed by a wide QRS. (*C*) DDD pacemaker. This dual-chamber pacemaker looks for a P wave; if no P wave is sensed, the pacemaker delivers a stimulus into the atrium. After a programmed AV delay, if no QRS is sensed, a second stimulus is delivered into the ventricle; the pacing spike is followed by a wide QRS.

intrinsic activity, a pacing stimulus may be delivered on the T wave, possibly inducing ventricular fibrillation. Newer pacemakers are capable of being synchronous and can vary their rate according to various physiologic parameters.

# ☐ PHYSIOLOGIC PACEMAKERS

Physiologic pacemakers are designed to maintain or increase cardiac output in a physiologic manner. They represent a significant advance in pacemaker technology when compared with earlier units.

First-generation pacemakers were single-chamber units designed to deliver impulses into one chamber (usually the ventricle); their purpose was simply to maintain heart rate. Second-generation dual-chamber pacemakers were designed to simulate the normal sequence of depolarization in the heart—a more physiologic approach. Dual-chamber pacemakers stimulate the atria and the ventricles in sequence, thereby preserving normal AV synchrony and the "atrial kick" that contributes to up to 20 to 30 percent of cardiac output.

Dual-chamber pacing units use two catheters, one in the right atrium and the other in the right ventricle. These pacers are programmed to function in the inhibited (demand) mode, although triggering is also incorporated into more sophisticated units. AV synchrony is preserved by sending an impulse first into the atrium to produce a P wave (if a P wave is not sensed); if a QRS is not sensed within a programmed AV delay, the generator will send another impulse into the ventricle to produce a QRS complex.

BOX 14-2 **Dual-Chamber Pacemaker Functions**

There are four easy ways to describe how a dual-chamber pacemaker is functioning:

1. **Inhibited function.** When both the intrinsic P waves and QRS complexes are sensed, both atrial and ventricular pacemaker outputs are inhibited. In other words, the pacemaker is not firing at all. Only the native cardiac rhythm is seen.
2. **AV synchronous function.** When both the intrinsic P waves and QRS complexes are not sensed, the atrial output is delivered. After a programmed AV delay, the ventricular output is delivered. In other words, the two chambers are stimulated in sequence to simulate normal AV synchrony. The native cardiac rhythm is not seen.
3. **P wave synchronous function.** When an intrinsic P wave is sensed, the pacemaker waits a period of time (the programmed AV delay) before it delivers a pacing stimulus into the ventricle. In other words, a native P wave is followed by a ventricular paced event.
4. **Atrial paced function.** When no intrinsic P wave is sensed, a pacing stimulus is delivered into the atrium. The impulse is conducted through the AV node into the ventricle to produce an intrinsic QRS complex. In other words, an atrial paced event is followed by a native QRS complex. Atrial pacing is used only if conduction through the AV node is intact.

Third-generation **rate-responsive** pacemakers represent a major leap in pacemaker technology. These single-chamber or dual-chamber units allow the rate of pacing to increase in response to physiologic demand. They are programmed to respond to features including activity, respirations, blood temperature, blood pH, and other parameters that are under investigation.

Candidates for dual-chamber pacing include patients who cannot tolerate the loss of AV synchrony associated with conventional VVI pacing (single-chamber ventricular demand pacing). These patients are most likely to experience the pacemaker syndrome—a cluster of symptoms (including dizziness, weakness, and lethargy) associated with loss of the "atrial kick" during VVI pacing.

**CLINICAL TIP**
Patients with chronic atrial fibrillation are not candidates for dual-chamber pacemakers. The fibrillating atria do not respond to atrial pacemaker output signals.

# ☐ MALFUNCTION

Thorough knowledge of each pacemaker's specific functions and parameters must precede any attempt to diagnose a pacemaker malfunction. A wide variety of pacemakers are available, and different combinations of features are used, so one should never assume that all pacemakers are alike.

Pacemaker malfunction results from abnormalities in sensing, firing, and/or capturing. Most of these problems can be traced to component failure, battery failure, or problems at the interface between the catheter tip and the heart.

**Note:** Some problems associated with newer DDD (dual-chamber) pacemakers are actually errors in interpretation (pseudomalfunction) rather than actual malfunction.

## SENSING MALFUNCTIONS

**Undersensing** is the most common cause of a failure to sense. The generator's sensitivity (mV) may be set too high (it is not sensitive enough and cannot "see" incoming signals), the voltage of the incoming signals may be too low (not unusual in patients with ischemic heart disease), or the lead is out of position. Also, oversensing (T waves, muscle artifact, etc.) may allow undersensing of appropriate (QRS) signals. Paced beats appear too early, too late, or not at all.

### Interventions for Undersensing
1. Increase the sensitivity of a temporary generator by turning the sensitivity or millivolt dial to a lower number (e.g., from 10 to 2); then observe for paced beats that appear on time.
2. Reprogram a permanent generator to increase the sensitivity (lower the mV setting).

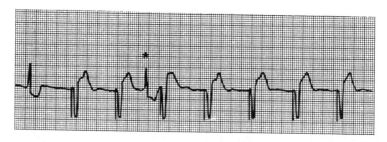

**FIGURE 14–10.** Undersensing. The pacemaker fires earlier than it should because it has not sensed the QRS complex *(asterisk)*. (From Beare, PG and Myers, JL: Principles and Practice of Adult Health Nursing. CV Mosby, St. Louis, 1990, p 798, with permission.)

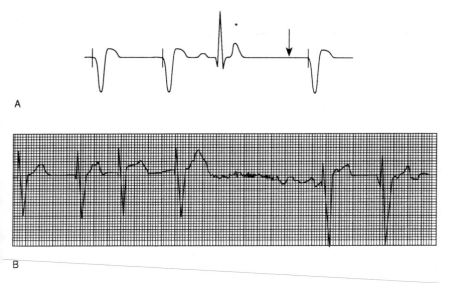

A

B

**FIGURE 14-11.** Oversensing. (*A*) The pacemaker is inhibited by a giant T wave (*asterisk*). Instead of firing on time (*arrow*), the pacemaker fires later than it should. (*B*) Muscle tremor artifact can be sensed inappropriately, which inhibits the pacemaker from firing.

3. Do an overpenetrated chest x-ray to check for lead position; reposition the pacing lead if necessary.

**Oversensing** means that the generator is too sensitive and is sensing the wrong signals (e.g., T waves instead of QRS complexes, or muscle tremor artifact). Oversensing can cause inhibition of the pacemaker impulse.

## Interventions for Oversensing
1. Decrease the sensitivity of a temporary generator by turning the sensitivity or millivolt dial to a higher number (e.g., from 2 to 5) until the unit starts to sense appropriately.
2. Convert a permanent pacemaker to fixed rate by placing a magnet over the generator site (the magnet will blind the sensing circuits).

   **Note:** This is a temporary maneuver designed to preserve pacing until the underlying problem is corrected.

3. Reprogram a permanent generator to decrease the sensitivity, or rarely change to the asynchronous mode.

**Inappropriate sensing** may lead to inhibition of the output signal. Exposure of a pacing unit to electromagnetic interference (e.g., from older-model microwave ovens, electrocautery devices, magnetic resonance imaging [MRI]) may result in inappropriate inhibition of the output signal.

BOX 14–3 **Pacemaker-Mediated Tachycardia**

Dual-chamber pacemakers (those with two leads implanted, one each in the atrium and ventricle) are sometimes associated with a unique dysrhythmia called pacemaker-mediated tachycardia (PMT). One of the most common precipitating events is a ventricular premature complex (VPC). As long as retrograde conduction is intact (the impulse can travel backward from the ventricle through the AV node), the abnormal impulse may be conducted retrogradely into the atria to produce a P wave. If the atrial lead senses the retrograde P wave, ventricular pacing via the ventricular lead will follow automatically after a programmed delay at the AV node. Each subsequent event (QRS followed by retrograde P) perpetuates the cycle. PMT can usually be abolished acutely by placing a magnet over the generator. Long-term prevention of PMT includes drugs to decrease atrioventricular conduction and reprogramming certain parameters of the pacemaker.

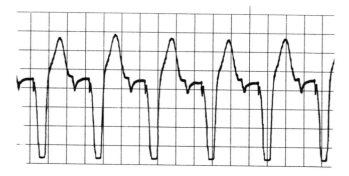

Note the retrograde P wave visible just after the T wave. Each time a retrograde P wave is sensed, ventricular pacing follows. If the cycle perpetuates itself, pacemaker-mediated tachycardia is the result. (From Kern, LS: Cardiac Critical Care Nursing. Aspen Publishers, Rockville, MD, 1988, p 235, with permission.)

## *Interventions for Inappropriate Sensing*
1. Avoid potential sources of electromagnetic interference.
2. Include information about potential sources of electromagnetic interference in the discharge planning instructions. Refer to manufacturer's instructions regarding environmental hazards (e.g., overhead transmission lines and welding equipment).

## Firing Malfunctions

**Failure to fire** means that a pacing spike fails to appear when it should. Failure to fire can result from depletion of the pacemaker battery, fracture of

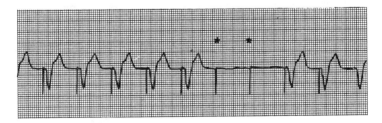

**FIGURE 14-12.** Failure to fire. The pacemaker spike does not appear when it should *(asterisk)*. (From Beare, PG and Myers JL: Principles and Practice of Adult Health Nursing. CV Mosby, St. Louis, 1990, p 798, with permission.)

the pacing catheter or its insulation, a disconnection somewhere within the system, or oversensing.

## Interventions for Failure to Fire

1. Tighten all connections in a temporary system.
2. Replace the battery in a temporary generator (wear gloves, turn the unit off during battery replacement, mark the generator indicating the date of a battery change).
3. Do an overpenetrated chest x-ray to detect lead wire fracture (may be difficult to detect).
4. Replace the pacing catheter.
5. Replace the battery in a permanent generator (requires reoperation).
6. Evaluate for oversensing.
7. Newer technology allows for impedance and/or electrogram to be evaluated through the pacer lead utilizing a special analyzer.

## CAPTURING MALFUNCTIONS

**Failure to capture** means that the expected waveform fails to appear after the pacing spike. Failure to capture is common with temporary pacemakers and often results from either migration of the catheter tip within the heart or loss of contact with the wall of the heart. In permanent pacemakers, failure to capture may occur with lead fracture or fibrosis at the lead tip causing exit block (inability of the impulse to enter the myocardium).

**FIGURE 14-13.** Failure to capture. On two occasions *(asterisks)* the pacemaker spike is not followed by a wide QRS complex. (From Beare, PG and Myers, JL: Principles and Practice of Adult Health Nursing. CV Mosby, St. Louis, 1990, p 798, with permission.)

## Interventions for Failure to Capture

1. Increase the milliamperes on a temporary generator until effective capture is achieved.
2. Do an overpenetrated chest x-ray to determine catheter position.
3. If the catheter is out of position, a *temporary* maneuver is to place the patient on his or her left side (gravity may allow the catheter to contact the endocardium).
4. Reposition the pacing catheter.
5. Use a bridging cable (or extension cable) to reduce traction on externalized pacing wires.
6. Reprogram a permanent generator.
7. Teach the patient about recommended postinsertion activity.

---

BOX 14-4 **Pacemaker Pearls**

- Insertion of a temporary pacing catheter into the heart can cause dysrhythmias. Be prepared to intervene with drugs or countershock or both.
- If defibrillation is required, turn off a temporary pacemaker to eliminate the risk of generator damage. If a permanent implant is present, avoid placing defibrillator paddles over the generator or close to it.
- Use a clear plastic cover over the face of a temporary generator to minimize the risk of damage if liquid is spilled on the controls.
- Insulate exposed metal. Use an unpowdered rubber glove.
- Protect exposed surgical wires. Cover them with a dressing, or place them within a protective sleeve or plastic tube.
- Minimize electrical hazards by ensuring that all electrical equipment is properly grounded.
- The patient with a pacemaker should not undergo MRI.
- Reduce the risk of catheter displacement by using a bridging cable between the generator and the external ends of a temporary pacing catheter. For femoral insertions, use a soft restraint on the ankle to prevent bending of the leg.
- Suspect perforation of the thin right ventricular wall by the pacing catheter if the patient begins to hiccough repeatedly or if a pericardial friction rub is heard. Do an overpenetrated chest x-ray to confirm catheter placement. If the diaphragm is being stimulated, the pacing catheter may have to be withdrawn and repositioned.
- Perforation of the interventricular septum by a stiff pacing catheter will cause a sudden change in the polarity of the paced QRS complex. When the right ventricle is stimulated during normal transvenous pacing, the spike is followed by a wide and negative QRS complex in lead $V_1$. If the catheter perforates the septum, the left ventricle will be stimulated first; the pacing spike will be followed by a wide and positive QRS complex in lead $V_1$.

BOX 14-4 (continued)

- Thrombosis and embolization from a pacing catheter is rare, but it can be fatal. Consider this possibility if the patient suddenly develops tachycardia, shortness of breath, or chest pain.
- Discharge teaching should include how to take the radial pulse (make sure that both patient and primary caregivers are able to demonstrate this skill), when to notify the physician (i.e., if the pulse falls below the preset pacing rate), what environmental hazards to avoid, and why postimplant follow-up is needed.

## ☐ KEY POINTS

- Most pacemakers are used when the heart rate is too slow. Antitachycardia pacemakers are occasionally used to slow or terminate the rate when it is too fast.
- The pulse generator contains replaceable batteries that generate the artificial electrical signal. The pacing catheter delivers the signal to the heart.
- Fixation devices on permanent pacing catheters help to ensure long-term contact with the heart muscle.
- Endocardial pacing means that the pacing catheter is inserted transvenously and is guided into the heart until it makes contact with the endocardium (inner surface). Epicardial pacing means that the pacing catheter is inserted using a transthoracic (or transxiphisternal) approach and is attached to the epicardium (outer surface).
- Because the pacing stimulus is delivered to only one ventricle, depolarization of the ventricles is sequential and prolonged, resulting in a QRS complex that is wider than normal.
- Transcutaneous pacing is used in emergency situations. The pacing stimulus is delivered to the heart through large pacing pads attached to the external chest wall.
- Sensing is the pacemaker's ability to process incoming signals.
- Firing is the pacemaker's ability to release a stimulus. Firing produces a pacing spike on the ECG.
- Capturing is the heart's ability to respond to a pacing stimulus. Capturing results in a P wave or QRS complex immediately after the pacing spike.
- The automatic interval is the pacing rate.
- The escape interval is the time between paced events and is usually the same as the automatic interval.

- Hysteresis is a programmable feature in single-chamber pacemakers that allows a slightly longer interval between a sensed intrinsic event and the first paced event.
- Milliamperes (mA) represent the strength of the output signal.
- Threshold is the minimum amount of current required to cause depolarization.
- Sensitivity (mV) is the ability of the generator to process or "see" incoming signals.
- The inhibited mode of pacing means that the pacemaker fires "on demand," or only when it does not sense an event (e.g., a QRS complex).
- The triggered mode means that the pacemaker is cued to fire after it senses an event.
- The asynchronous mode means that the pacemaker fires at a preset fixed rate; sensing is absent.
- Physiologic pacemakers (e.g., DDD) preserve normal AV synchrony and are designed to preserve the "atrial kick." Nonphysiologic pacemakers (e.g., VVI) are unable to preserve normal AV synchrony.
- Rate-responsive pacemakers control rate in response to physiologic demand by sensing selected parameters such as activity and blood pH.
- Failure to sense means that paced beats appear too early, too late, or not at all.
- Pacemaker-mediated tachycardia is associated with dual-chamber pacing units.
- Failure to fire is recognized by the absence of a scheduled pacing spike.
- Failure to capture means that the pacing spike is not followed by a P wave or QRS complex.

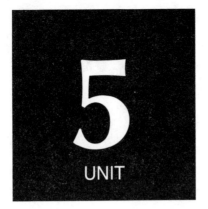

**5**

UNIT

# MYOCARDIAL INFARCTION

**CHAPTER 15**
Myocardial Infarction

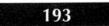

# Chapter

# 15

# MYOCARDIAL INFARCTION

The diagnosis of myocardial infarction (MI) is based on the patient's **clinical history**, serum **cardiac enzymes,** and the **12-lead electrocardiogram (ECG).** A single ECG, however, provides limited information about a complex picture. For an accurate diagnosis and evaluation of myocardial ischemia, injury, and infarction, **serial ECGs** must be obtained.

## ☐ ECG CHANGES OF ISCHEMIA, INJURY, AND INFARCTION

### ISCHEMIA

Myocardial ischemia denotes a temporary, reversible reduction of blood supply to heart muscle and is the earliest manifestation of reduced coronary blood flow. Ischemia is represented by **T wave changes** on the ECG. The normally upright, asymmetrical T wave becomes deeply inverted and symmetrical. This represents a **primary T wave change** and should be differentiated from the asymmetrical secondary T wave change associated with "digitalis effect" and strain (see Chapter 20). T wave inversion is usually seen during episodes of acute ischemia but may not show up for hours or days after the initial event. Serial ECGs obtained periodically (minutes to hours after the initial ECG) may be necessary to document myocardial ischemia, injury, or infarction.

### Pseudonormalization of the T Wave

Occasionally, inverted T waves may persist on serial ECGs owing to previous myocardial damage. In the patient with preexisting T wave inversion from a past event, acute ischemia may be represented by reversal to a normal,

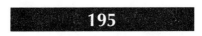

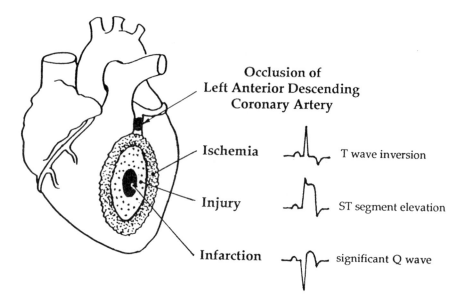

**FIGURE 15-1.** ECG changes of acute MI. In this example, occlusion of the left anterior descending coronary artery results in ischemia, injury, and infarction of heart muscle. ECG evidence of tissue damage is reflected in the T wave, ST segment, and initial QRS deflection (a significant Q wave develops). (Adapted from Lipman, BC and Lipman, BS: ECG Pocket Guide. Year Book Medical Publishers, Chicago, 1987, p 98, with permission.)

upright T wave on the ECG, a situation called **pseudonormalization** of the T wave. If previous 12-lead ECGs are available, they should always be evaluated in conjunction with the clinical history.

## INJURY

Myocardial injury results from an acute, prolonged reduction in blood supply to the myocardium. It is reversible if blood flow to areas of jeopardized myocardium is restored before tissue death occurs. Injury is represented by **ST segment changes** (elevation or depression) on the ECG.

**ST segment elevation** occurs during subepicardial injury (injury confined to the outer ventricular wall), often appearing within minutes to hours after the acute event. The ST segment is displaced upward from the baseline and its shape is "coved" or convex. The J point (at the beginning of the ST segment) is also elevated. This injury pattern represents reduced blood supply through a major epicardial coronary artery supplying oxygen to a large portion of the heart's outer surface. Two important causes of acute obstruction include atherosclerosis with sudden clot formation and, less commonly, coronary artery spasm. Coronary artery spasm (also termed variant or Prinzmetal's

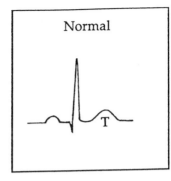

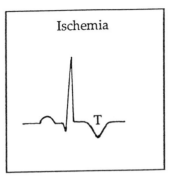

**FIGURE 15–2.** Acute myocardial ischemia. A normal T wave is upright, but ischemia causes symmetrical T wave inversion.

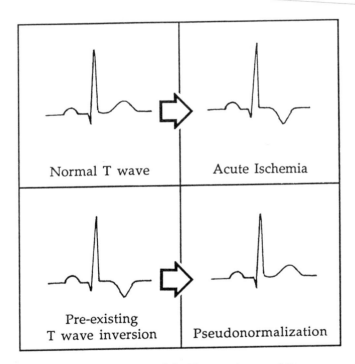

Normal T wave            Acute Ischemia

Pre-existing
T wave inversion       Pseudonormalization

**FIGURE 15–3.** Pseudonormalization of the T wave. A normal T wave may develop during an episode of acute ischemia in the patient with preexisting T wave inversion. Compare this "pseudonormalization" with the T wave inversion typically associated with acute ischemia. Old ECGs must be compared to current ECGs in order to correctly diagnose—or rule out—ischemia.

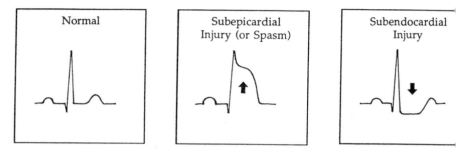

**FIGURE 15-4.** Acute myocardial injury. The ST segment is normally isoelectric. Subepicardial injury causes ST segment elevation, while subendocardial injury causes ST segment depression.

angina) usually lasts for only a few minutes, and when it resolves, the ST segment normally returns to the baseline.

**ST segment depression** occurs during subendocardial injury (injury confined to the inner ventricular wall). The innermost portion of the heart (endocardium) is perfused by small penetrating branches from the superficial epicardial coronary arteries. Its relatively poor perfusion makes the subendocardium the first area of myocardium to sustain injury when blood flow is compromised. If the blood supply is restored in time, the ST segment depression indicative of subendocardial injury may resolve. If blood flow is not restored in time, irreversible muscle damage may occur. This is called non–Q wave, or subendocardial, MI (see p 209).

ST segment depression is a clinical indicator of coronary artery disease during stress testing. The morphology of the ST segment depression (magnitude and slope) during exercise and the duration of ST segment depression after exercise are important criteria in assessing the severity of coronary artery disease (see p 240).

## INFARCTION

Myocardial infarction denotes irreversible death of heart muscle due to prolonged coronary artery occlusion. The classic ECG clue to infarction is the appearance of **significant Q waves** in leads representing the area of damage.

Abnormal Q waves represent electrically silent areas of infarcted heart muscle. The electrical forces in the heart travel through the "dead" (infarcted) area of myocardium. ECG electrodes "look through" this silent area of infarction and record only those electrical forces moving through undamaged muscle. The appearance of significant Q waves may be immediate or may lag behind other changes of acute MI by hours to days.

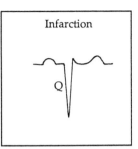

**FIGURE 15-5.** The Q wave of myocardial infarction. An abnormal Q wave denotes myocardial tissue death.

**CLINICAL TIP**
**Insignificant Q waves** are small Q waves—usually less than 25 percent of the height of the adjacent R wave—that may be found normally in leads I, aVL, $V_5$, and $V_6$. They result from the normal process of septal depolarization (see p 53). **Significant Q waves** (also called pathological) are abnormal Q waves that are deeper than 25 percent of the height of the adjacent R wave and greater than 0.04 second in duration.

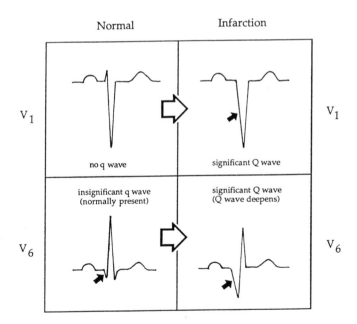

**FIGURE 15-6.** Significant Q waves. Lead $V_1$ does not normally record a Q wave; a significant Q wave may develop during infarction. Lead $V_6$ normally records an insignificant Q wave; infarction may cause the Q wave to deepen and widen.

BOX 15–1  **Summary of ECG Changes in Ischemia, Injury, Infarction**

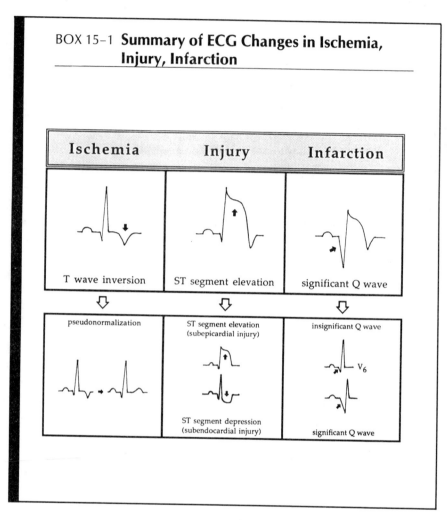

| Ischemia | Injury | Infarction |
|---|---|---|
| T wave inversion | ST segment elevation | significant Q wave |
| pseudonormalization | ST segment elevation (subepicardial injury) | insignificant Q wave |
| | ST segment depression (subendocardial injury) | significant Q wave |

# ☐ LOCALIZING ISCHEMIA, INJURY, AND INFARCTION

Areas of ischemia, injury, or infarction can usually be localized through careful assessment of a 12-lead ECG. Usually those leads oriented directly over an area of damage will reveal acute ECG changes (significant Q waves, ST segment elevation or depression, and T wave inversion), whereas leads "looking at" the surrounding healthy tissue will appear normal. ECG leads can be grouped to help localize the changes.

## BOX 15-2 **Analyzing Lead Groups**

Leads may be grouped according to the surface of the heart that they represent. ECG evidence of myocardial ischemia, injury, or infarction can be determined by analyzing changes that occur in leads oriented over or representing that area of the heart.

- **Anterior leads:**     $V_1$, $V_2$, $V_3$, $V_4$
- **Septal leads:**      $V_1$, $V_2$
- **Lateral leads:**      I, aVL, $V_5$, $V_6$
- **High lateral leads:**  I, aVL
- **Inferior leads:**     II, III, aVF
- **Posterior leads:**    $V_1$, $V_2$ (**Note:** Leads $V_1$ and $V_2$ are oriented opposite the posterior surface; they record mirror-image ECG changes in the presence of posterior damage.)

**Note:**  Lead aVR is not included in this list because it is rarely used in the diagnosis of acute MI.

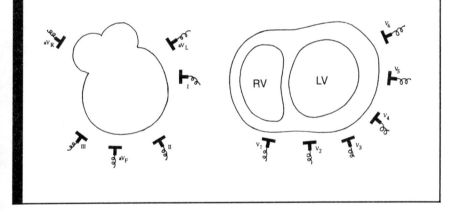

## ANTERIOR WALL MYOCARDIAL INFARCTION

Damage to the anterior surface of the left ventricle usually results from occlusion of the left anterior descending coronary artery. ECG changes are usually observed in anterior leads $V_1$ through $V_4$. Additionally, the R wave voltage observed in these chest leads may decrease in association with infarction. Because R waves reflect electrical forces moving through living heart muscle toward a recording electrode, *loss of R waves* in these leads (called poor R wave progression) may represent tissue death.

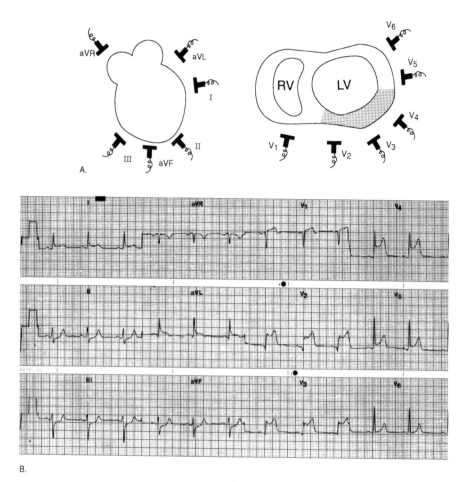

**FIGURE 15-7.** Anterior wall myocardial infarction. (*A*) AWMI usually causes ECG changes in chest leads $V_1$ through $V_4$ (LV, left ventricle; RV, right ventricle). (*B*) ST segment elevation is present in leads $V_1$ through $V_6$ as well as in leads I and aVL. Q waves are beginning to form in leads $V_1$ through $V_4$. Since ST segment elevation is present in the lateral leads (I, aVL, $V_5$, and $V_6$), the description "anterolateral wall MI" also applies. (*B* From Lipman, BC and Lipman, BS: ECG Pocket Guide. Year Book Medical Publishers, Chicago, 1987, p 182, with permission.)

## LATERAL WALL MYOCARDIAL INFARCTION

If occlusion of the circumflex coronary artery (or, less commonly, the right coronary artery) is present, damage to the lateral surface of the left ventricle may be reflected in leads I, aVL, $V_5$, and $V_6$.

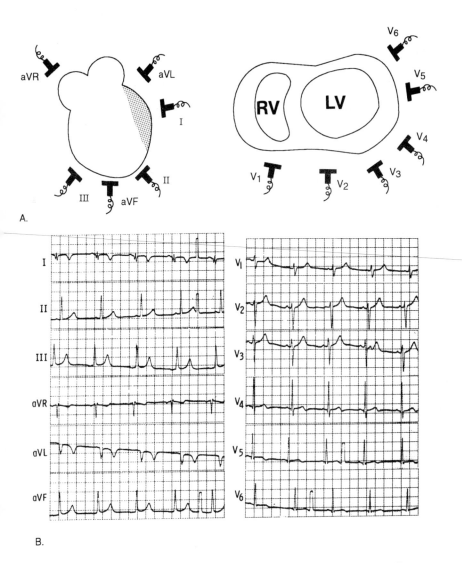

**FIGURE 15-8.** Lateral wall myocardial infarction. (*A*) Lateral wall MI usually causes ECG changes in chest leads $V_5$ and $V_6$ and in leads I and aVL (LV, left ventricle; RV, right ventricle). (*B*) Q waves and inverted T waves are present in leads I and aVL. (*B* From Chung, EK: Electrocardiography: Practical Applications and Vectorial Principles, ed 3. Appleton & Lange, CT, 1985, p 121, with permission.)

## INFERIOR WALL MYOCARDIAL INFARCTION

Damage to the inferior (diaphragmatic) surface of the heart usually results from occlusion of the right coronary artery (or, less commonly, the circumflex coronary artery). The ECG reveals acute changes in inferior leads II, III, and aVF. In up to one third of inferior wall MIs, the right ventricle may also be involved, and ECG changes of right ventricular infarction will be present (Box 15–3).

---

### BOX 15-3 **Diagnosis of Right Ventricular Infarction**

The ECG changes of right ventricular infarction may be seen in lead $V_1$ or in unconventional **right-sided chest leads** $V_{3R}$ and $V_{4R}$. $V_R$ leads are created by placing chest leads $V_3$ through $V_6$ over the *right* precordium (rather than the left). $V_R$ leads are not included as part of a conventional 12-lead ECG, but they may be created when a closer look at right-sided ECG changes is desired. ST segment elevation in right chest leads $V_{3R}$ and $V_{4R}$ confirms acute right ventricular infarction.

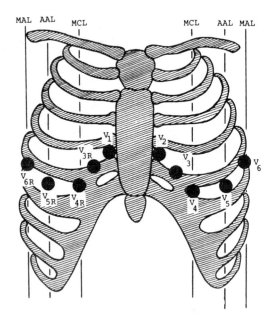

(From Chung, EK: Electrocardiography: Practical Applications with Vectorial Principles, ed 3, Appleton & Lange, Norwalk, Ct, 1985, p 21, with permission.)

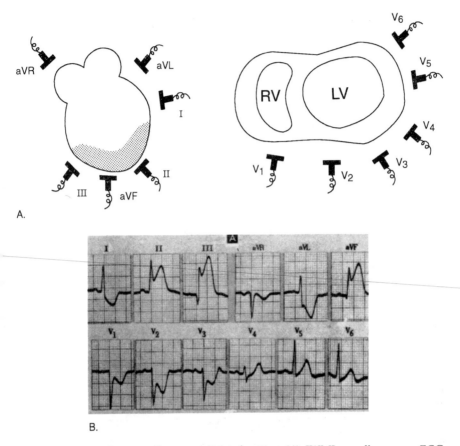

A.

B.

**FIGURE 15-9.** Inferior wall myocardial infarction. (A) IWMI usually causes ECG changes in leads II, III, and aVF (LV, left ventricle; RV, right ventricle). (B) There is marked ST segment elevation in leads II, III, and aVF; Q waves are beginning to form in these leads. The ST segment depression observed in leads I, aVL, and $V_1$ through $V_3$ is called a reciprocal (or mirror-image) change (see text). (B From Lipman, BC and Lipman, BS: ECG Pocket Guide. Year Book Medical Publishers, Chicago, 1987, p 181, with permission.)

## POSTERIOR WALL MYOCARDIAL INFARCTION

Posterior wall MI may be seen in conjunction with inferior wall MI and is usually caused by occlusion of the right coronary artery. Because there are no conventional leads placed directly over the posterior wall of the heart, ECG evidence of infarction must be inferred from opposing leads, primarily chest leads $V_1$ and $V_2$. These leads, which are oriented *opposite* the site of infarction, may reveal taller-than-expected R waves, ST segment depression, and upright T waves.

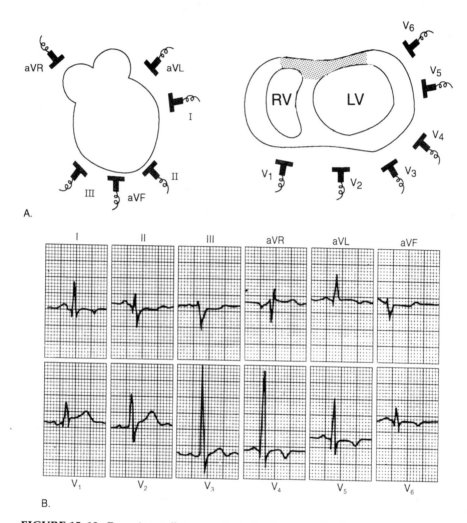

**FIGURE 15–10.** Posterior wall myocardial infarction. (A) PWMI usually causes ECG changes in leads $V_1$ and $V_2$. Since these leads are oriented opposite the area of damage, ECG changes are the opposite of what is expected in leads oriented directly over the area of damage (LV, left ventricle; RV, right ventricle). (B) The R wave is taller than expected, and the T waves are upright in leads $V_1$ through $V_3$. (B from Wilson, RF: Critical Care Manual: Applied Physiology and Principles of Therapy, ed 2. FA Davis, Philadelphia, 1992, p 80, with permission.)

# ☐ EVOLUTION OF ACUTE MI AND RECIPROCAL ECG CHANGES

## EVOLUTION

Evolution of the infarction pattern typically involves the development of acute ECG changes with gradual reversion of the ST segments and T waves back to normal over time. During acute obstruction of a coronary artery, the ECG findings of ischemia (T wave inversion), injury (ST segment elevation or depression), and infarction (significant Q waves) are usually seen in leads representing the area of damage. However, the period of time during which these ECG changes are found is often highly variable. In fact, one, two, all three— or none—of these ECG findings may be recorded during an "evolving" MI. Usually, there is initial acute ST segment elevation (or depression) with or without T wave inversion. Significant Q waves usually form within the first few hours, but this time period is highly variable. If thrombolytic therapy or coronary angioplasty is performed in the acute setting, and if blood flow is successfully restored (i.e., if myocardial tissue death is prevented), the ST segment elevation or depression may subside and significant Q waves may not form.

Clearly, the clinical history and interpretation of *serial* tracings are important in evaluating an evolving acute MI. With the exception of the significant Q wave (sometimes a permanent fixture on the tracing), ECG changes associated with acute MI (ST segment and T wave changes) may resolve over a period of days, weeks, or months.

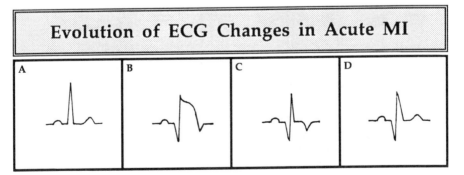

**Evolution of ECG Changes in Acute MI**

| A | B | C | D |
|---|---|---|---|

FIGURE 15-11. Evolution of ECG changes in acute MI. (*A*) Normal. (*B*) Acute changes (significant Q wave, ST segment elevation, and T wave inversion). (*C*) Resolving (the ST segment has returned to the baseline, but T wave inversion and the significant Q wave remain). (*D*) Stable (the T wave is upright again; the significant Q wave remains).

## RECIPROCAL CHANGES

Sometimes during acute MI, leads oriented opposite the area of infarction may reveal reciprocal (or mirror-image) changes. In other words, the injury pattern of ST segment elevation may be seen in one group of leads, while reciprocal ST segment depression may be seen in the group of leads oriented opposite the area of injury. For example, acute *inferior* MI with associated ST segment elevation in the inferior leads (II, III, and aVF) may be accompanied by **reciprocal** ST segment depression in the lateral leads (I and aVL) or in the anterior leads ($V_1$ through $V_4$). Similarly, *anterior* infarction with ST segment elevation in the anterior leads ($V_1$ through $V_4$) may be associated with **reciprocal** ST segment depression in the opposing inferior leads (II, III, and aVF). Reciprocal changes usually resolve over time.

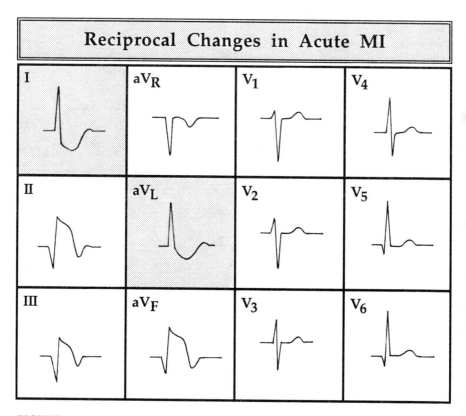

### Reciprocal Changes in Acute MI

FIGURE 15–12. Reciprocal changes in acute MI. In this example of IWMI, typical ECG changes are noted in leads II, III, and aVF. Reciprocal changes (primarily ST segment depression) are recorded in leads oriented opposite the area of damage (I and aVL).

# ☐ Q WAVE VERSUS NON–Q WAVE MI

The longer the heart muscle is deprived of oxygen, the more widespread the area of tissue death. The first area of myocardium to succumb during acute coronary occlusion is usually the subendocardium, the poorly perfused area of heart muscle farthest away from the larger, surface epicardial coronary artery. Ultimately, muscle necrosis may extend from the subendocardium to the subepicardium, reflecting damage that extends through the entire thickness of the heart muscle.

Usually, if the acute MI affects only the subendocardium, a significant Q wave will not develop in the ECG. This type of infarction is termed a **non–Q wave**, or **subendocardial, MI.** On the other hand, if the infarction affects the

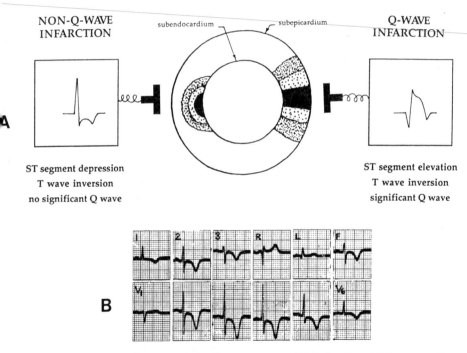

**FIGURE 15–13.** Non–Q wave versus Q wave myocardial infarction. (*A*) in a non–Q wave MI, muscle damage is confined to the subendocardium. In a Q wave MI, muscle damage extends from the subendocardium to the subepicardium. (Adapted from Lipman, BC and Lipman, BS: ECG Pocket Guide. Year Book Medical Publishers, Chicago, 1987, p 106, with permission.) (*B*) Non–Q wave MI. Widespread ST segment depression and T wave inversion is visible in the limb and chest leads, but no significant Q waves have developed. (From Marriott, HJL: Practical Electrocardiography, ed 7. Williams & Wilkins, Baltimore, 1983, p 387, with permission.)

entire thickness of the ventricular wall—from the subendocardium to the subepicardium—an abnormal Q wave will usually develop on the ECG. This type of infarction is termed a **Q wave,** or **transmural,** MI.

Non–Q wave MIs usually imply less myocardial tissue death than transmural MIs, and they are accompanied by fewer complications and a reduced mortality during the initial hospitalization. These infarctions usually result when a coronary artery occludes and then suddenly reopens to reperfuse the heart muscle. Even though non–Q wave MIs are usually smaller and less troublesome during the acute period, they may develop into transmural MIs later. The majority of patients with initial non–Q wave MIs may still have a severely blocked coronary artery that may reocclude within the next 3 to 6 months, resulting in a Q wave MI (transmural). Clearly, patients experiencing non–Q wave MI represent a specific group at high risk for future cardiac events. They must be very closely evaluated for sudden extension of the infarct within the first few months after the initial event.

**CLINICAL TIP**

Additional ECG findings that may help in distinguishing Q wave from non–Q wave MIs:

1. ST segment depression is seen more commonly with non–Q wave (subendocardial) MI.
2. ST segment elevation is seen more commonly with Q wave (transmural) MI, unless the MI is aborted with thrombolytic therapy or acute coronary angioplasty; if recanalization (restoration of blood flow) is successful, ST segment displacement will subside.
3. T wave inversion may be seen in both types of infarctions.

**CLINICAL TIP**

The patient experiencing a non–Q wave MI is most at risk after the first few days. All complaints of pain must be carefully evaluated because they may represent extension of the infarct.

# ☐ INITIATION OF THROMBOLYTIC THERAPY

With the advent of thrombolytic agents, acute coronary artery occlusions (the majority of which are caused by thrombus superimposed on atherosclerosis) can often be opened **(recanalized),** resulting in preservation of heart muscle. Many studies have shown a reduction in morbidity and mortality with the *early* use of acute thrombolytic therapy. Thrombolytic agents act by dissolving fresh coronary thrombus and reestablishing coronary blood flow to previously compromised muscle. The cost and potentially serious side effects associated with these potent agents make the indications and contraindications for their use very important.

## INDICATIONS FOR THROMBOLYTIC THERAPY

1. ST segment elevation in two or more leads associated with acute chest pain
2. Time between onset of chest pain to initiation of therapy less than 24 hours (optimal time to initiate therapy is less than 6 hours, and *the earlier the better*).

## CONTRAINDICATIONS TO THROMBOLYTIC THERAPY

1. Stroke within the previous 1 to 2 years (because of the risk of intracerebral bleeding)
2. Major surgery within the previous 2 weeks
3. History of gastrointestinal bleeding
4. Severe hypertension
5. History of coagulopathy or tendency toward bleeding

# ☐ COMPLICATIONS OF ACUTE MI

Complications associated with acute MI depend on both the location and the size of the infarction. Small infarctions may not produce clinically significant complications, whereas large MIs can result in life-threatening electromechanical problems.

Serious **mechanical** complications of infarction include cardiogenic shock (often associated with anterior wall MI), free wall ventricular rupture (possibly creating cardiac tamponade), septal wall rupture (creating an acute ventricular septal defect), and papillary muscle rupture (resulting in acute mitral regurgitation).

Equally serious **electrical** complications of infarction are observed frequently both during and after the acute event. These dysrhythmias with their associated findings and treatments are summarized here (see Appendix A for specific drug dosages):

1. **Sinus bradycardia.** Seen often with inferior wall MI

   **Treatment:** Atropine may be given for **symptomatic** bradycardia. Temporary pacing may be required.

   **Note:** Acceleration of rate should be undertaken cautiously to prevent extension of the infarct (caused by a rate-related increase in oxygen demand).

2. **Junctional rhythm, accelerated junctional rhythm.** Seen with inferior wall MI

   **Treatment:** Atropine may be given in the presence of a symptomatic bradycardia. Pacing may be necessary.

**Note:** Investigate the cause of an accelerated junctional rhythm, as it may be associated with digitalis.

3. **Atrial premature complexes (APCs).** Often seen in association with heart failure

   **Treatment:** Usually unnecessary

4. **Atrial fibrillation, atrial flutter**

   **Treatment:** Digoxin may be given. Also, careful administration of beta blockers or calcium channel blockers is appropriate to slow ventricular rate. Cardioversion may be necessary if the patient is unstable.

   **Note:** Calcium channel blockers and beta blockers can cause significant hypotension.

5. **Ventricular premature complexes (VPCs).** Commonly observed during acute MI; treatment based on evaluation of the clinical situation

   **Treatment:** Xylocaine, procainamide, quinidine, phenytoin, and bretylium are among the drug treatment choices.

   **Note:** Prophylactic antidysrhythmic drug therapy may be considered for some patients in the acute setting.

6. **Ventricular tachycardia (VT).** Often a life-threatening prelude to ventricular fibrillation (VF)

   **Treatment:** Xylocaine, procainamide, and bretylium may be given. Precordial thump may be necessary (for a witnessed VT only), followed by defibrillation if patient is hemodynamically unstable. Cardioversion may be required for sustained VT.

   **Note:** Cardioversion may be successful at lower energy levels than are usually required to terminate VF.

7. **Ventricular fibrillation.** Most common during the first few hours after the acute event

   **Treatment:** Immediate defibrillation and administration of epinephrine, xylocaine, procainamide, and bretylium may be needed.

8. **Accelerated idioventricular rhythm (AIVR).** May be seen with acute coronary reperfusion and inferior wall MI

   **Treatment:** There is usually none; atropine may be used to increase the sinus rate to override the AIVR. Xylocaine is not used to suppress AIVR unless it degenerates into VT.

   **Note:** AIVR is often a transient dysrhythmia that produces no untoward clinical symptoms.

9. **First-degree atrioventricular (AV) block.** Often associated with inferior wall MI

    **Treatment:** Usually no treatment is necessary unless there is associated block below the bundle of His (seen more often with large anterior wall MIs).

    **Note:** Symptoms associated with first-degree AV block result from the underlying rate and not from the AV block itself.

10. **Second-degree AV block, type I (Mobitz type I, or Wenckebach phenomenon).** Seen commonly after inferior MI; usually transient

    **Treatment:** None is usually needed, but watch for widening of the QRS complex, which may represent an associated intraventricular block (possibly heralding the development of a higher-degree AV block).

    **Note:** Symptoms that occur in association with type I block are usually due to a slow underlying sinus rate rather than to the block itself. Symptoms may also occur if beats are dropped frequently.

11. **Second-degree AV block, type II (Mobitz type II).** Most often associated with anterior wall MI and a large amount of myocardial damage; may progress to third-degree AV block

    **Treatment:** Atropine for an associated symptomatic bradycardia. Temporary pacing followed by permanent pacing because of the tendency to progress to complete AV block later.

    **Note:** Symptoms are rare unless the underlying sinus rate is slow and/or the frequency of dropped beats produces significant pauses on the ECG.

12. **Third-degree (complete) AV block**

    **Treatment:** Temporary pacemaker followed by permanent pacemaker is usually indicated.

    **Note:** Complete AV block with a narrow–QRS-complex escape rhythm (junctional escape pacemaker) may not require a pacemaker. It is often seen during inferior wall MI.

13. **Fascicular blocks (hemiblocks).** Left anterior fascicular block occurs commonly and may be associated with right bundle branch block (RBBB). Left posterior fascicular block, on the other hand, is uncommon and usually does not occur unless a large amount of myocardial damage is present.

    **Treatment:** Depending on the location of the infarct and severity of heart block, temporary and/or permanent pacemakers may be indicated.

**Note:**    Bifascicular block (two of three fascicles blocked, as in RBBB and left anterior fascicular block) may progress to complete heart block, especially if it is associated with first-degree AV block.

## CLINICAL TIP

- Heart failure can occur with any MI, but anterior wall MI is most often associated with *severe* degrees of heart failure (including pulmonary edema and cardiogenic shock) because of the larger amount of myocardial damage usually present.
- Dysrhythmias can occur with any infarct. Life-threatening dysrhythmias (e.g., VF) are most likely to occur within the first few hours after the acute event.
- Bundle branch blocks are most likely to occur in association with anterior wall MI.
- AV blocks and AIVR are most likely to occur in association with inferior wall MI.
- Inferior wall MI may be accompanied by posterior wall involvement, and vice versa. Damage in these locations may be associated with papillary muscle dysfunction and acute mitral regurgitation.

## KEY POINTS

- Accurate evaluation of myocardial ischemia, injury, and infarction requires examination of *serial* ECGs.
- Ischemia denotes temporary, reversible reduction of blood supply to the heart muscle. It is reflected by T wave inversion on the ECG.
- Acute ischemia may cause normalization of the T wave (instead of T wave inversion) in patients with preexisting T wave inversion. This is called pseudonormalization of the T wave.
- Injury denotes prolonged, but reversible, reduction of blood supply to the heart muscle. It is reflected by either elevation or depression of the ST segment on the ECG.
- ST segment elevation is associated with subepicardial injury, whereas ST segment depression is associated with subendocardial injury.
- Infarction denotes irreversible death of heart muscle. It may produce significant (pathologic) Q waves on the ECG.
- ECG changes associated with acute MI (significant Q waves, ST segment elevation, and T wave inversion) are most prominent in leads oriented over the area of damage.
- $V_R$ leads are used to assess right-sided cardiac changes.
- The time when the classic ECG changes of infarction appear is highly variable. Acute ST segment elevation is often the first indicator, followed by T wave inversion and development of significant Q waves.

- ECG (ST segment and T wave) changes associated with acute MI usually resolve over time.
- Reciprocal changes are mirror-image ECG changes sometimes observed in leads oriented opposite the area of damage.
- A non–Q wave infarction reflects damage confined to the subendocardium.
- A Q wave infarction reflects transmural tissue damage.
- Patients who have experienced a non–Q wave MI are at risk for extension of the infarct within the first few months after the initial event.
- Thrombolytics ("clot busters") administered as soon as possible after the onset of an acute MI may prevent tissue death by restoring blood flow through a coronary vessel.

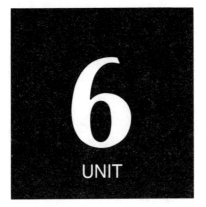

# 6
## UNIT

# MISCELLANEOUS
# CONDITIONS

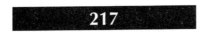

# Chapter

# 16

# CHAMBER ENLARGEMENT

Chamber enlargement may involve the atria, the ventricles, or both. It implies either **dilatation** (an increase in the internal diameter of the cardiac chamber) or actual **hypertrophy** (thickening) of the chamber walls. Chamber enlargement (whether due to dilatation or to true hypertrophy) is often called "hypertrophy."

> **Note:** Chamber enlargement may reflect either dilatation or hypertrophy.

Although chamber enlargement is suggested by numerous ECG clues, it is usually impossible to differentiate dilatation from hypertrophy using the ECG alone. Diagnostic tools such as echocardiography are usually required to pinpoint the true nature of chamber enlargement.

## ☐ ATRIAL CHAMBER ENLARGEMENT

**Atrial chamber enlargement** (also called **atrial abnormality** or **atrial hypertrophy**) is caused by clinical conditions that either increase atrial work or impose a volume overload on the right or left atrium. It often accompanies ventricular chamber enlargement. Common causes of atrial chamber enlargement are stenotic or regurgitant valves, congenital heart defects, and chronic pulmonary disease (which affects the right atrium).

*ECG clues to atrial chamber enlargement are reflected by changes in the P wave.* Enlargement of the right or left atrium will cause a change in the height (voltage) or width of the P wave as well as a shift in the P wave axis. These changes are best observed in inferior limb leads II, III, and aVF and in precordial leads $V_1$ and $V_2$. Normally a biphasic P wave (deflected above and below the baseline) is observed in leads $V_1$ and $V_2$. The initial (positive) portion of the

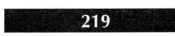

P wave reflects depolarization forces recorded from the right atrium, whereas the terminal (negative) portion reflects depolarization forces recorded from the left atrium. If right or left atrial chamber enlargement is present, one of these P wave components will be exaggerated.

> *Note: Atrial chamber enlargement causes P wave changes.*

## ECG CLUES TO RIGHT ATRIAL ABNORMALITY (OR ENLARGEMENT)

1. Tall, peaked P wave (greater than 2.5 mm in height) in inferior leads II, III, and aVF (also called P pulmonale)
2. Tall initial upstroke of the P wave in lead $V_1$ with a small terminal negative deflection (reflects exaggerated depolarization forces in the right atrium)
3. P wave width remaining normal

> *Note: Right atrial abnormality (enlargement or hypertrophy) is also called P pulmonale.*

## ECG CLUES TO LEFT ATRIAL ABNORMALITY (OR ENLARGEMENT)

1. Notched or m-shaped P wave in leads I, II, and aVL (also called P mitrale)
2. Small initial upstroke of the P wave in lead $V_1$ with a deep terminal negative deflection (reflects exaggerated depolarization forces in the left atrium)
3. P wave width wider than normal (greater than 0.11 second)

> *Note: Left atrial abnormality (enlargement or hypertrophy) is also called P mitrale.*

## ☐ VENTRICULAR CHAMBER ENLARGEMENT

**Ventricular chamber enlargement** often accompanies atrial abnormality and is caused by clinical conditions that either increase ventricular work or impose a volume overload on the ventricle. Common causes are stenotic or regurgitant valves and increased afterload (or increased vascular tone, as in systemic or pulmonary hypertension).

*ECG clues to ventricular chamber enlargement are reflected by changes in the QRS complex, ST segment, and T wave.* Enlargement of the right or left ventricle

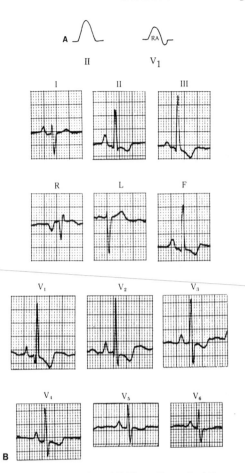

**FIGURE 16–1.** Right atrial abnormality. (*A*) The tall, peaked P wave illustrated in lead II is called P-pulmonale. In lead $V_1$ the tall initial upstroke of the P wave reflects right atrial enlargement. (*B*) Note the tall, peaked P waves evident in the inferior leads. P waves in the right-sided chest leads are also peaked. (From Conover, MB: Understanding Electrocardiography: Arrhythmias and the 12-Lead ECG, ed 5. CV Mosby, St. Louis, 1988, p. 311, with permission.)

will cause a change in the height (voltage) and width of the QRS complex, as well as a shift in the QRS axis. Changes in the QRS axis are best observed in the limb leads, but changes in QRS voltage and width are most obvious in chest leads $V_1$ through $V_6$. ST segment and T wave changes usually accompany changes in QRS voltage. These ST segment and T wave alterations result from abnormal ventricular depolarization and are called **secondary repolarization changes.**

Normally, electrical forces from the larger left ventricle are dominant, causing the majority of the depolarization forces to travel away from right chest leads ($V_1$ and $V_2$). The resulting QRS complex is predominantly negative

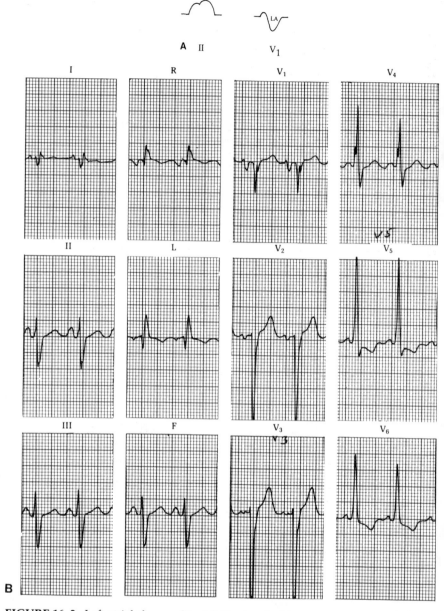

**FIGURE 16–2.** Left atrial abnormality. (*A*) The notched P wave illustrated in lead II is called P-mitrale. In lead $V_1$ the deep terminal deflection of the P wave reflects left atrial enlargement. (*B*) Note the notched P waves evident in the inferior leads. P waves in right-sided chest leads exhibit a deep terminal deflection. (From Conover, MB: Understanding Electrocardiography: Arrhythmias and the 12-Lead ECG, ed 5. CV Mosby, St. Louis, 1988, p. 309, with permission.)

## BOX 16–1 ECG Changes of Atrial Hypertrophy/ Enlargement

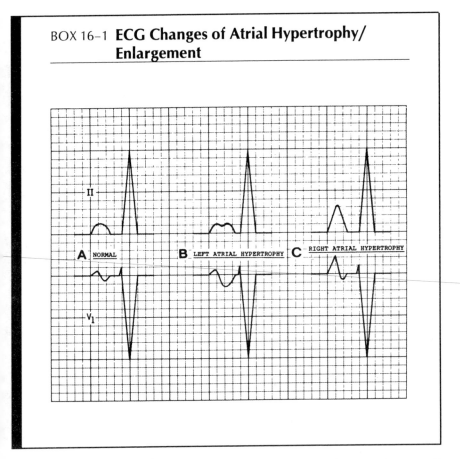

P wave changes associated with right and left atrial enlargement (compared to normal) in leads II and $V_1$. (From Chung, EK: Electrocardiography: Practical Applications with Vectorial Principles, ed 3. Appleton & Lange, Norwalk, CT, 1985, p 44, with permission.)

in lead $V_1$ and positive in lead $V_6$ (see normal R wave progression, p 51). Chamber enlargement either reverses or exaggerates normal QRS morphology and voltage in the chest leads.

**Note:** *Ventricular chamber enlargement causes changes in the QRS complex, ST segment, and T wave.*

## ECG CLUES TO RIGHT VENTRICULAR ENLARGEMENT

If right ventricular enlargement is present, normal left-sided dominance is blunted by exaggerated forces generated from the right ventricle. The QRS complex in lead $V_1$ becomes positive with a taller-than-expected R wave, and the QRS complex in lead $V_6$ becomes more negative with a deeper-than-expected S wave. Normal R wave progression is delayed in left chest leads (e.g., leads $V_5$ and $V_6$).

## ECG Criteria

1. Right axis deviation: The QRS axis is between $+90°$ and $+180°$ (the axis usually shifts because right ventricular muscle mass increases significantly).
2. The height (or voltage) of the QRS complex is increased in leads that record right ventricular forces.
   - The height of the R wave exceeds the depth of the S wave in lead $V_1$.
   - The R wave is greater than 7 mm in lead $V_1$ and greater than 5 mm in lead aVR.
   - The S wave in lead $V_1$ is less than 2 mm.
3. The negative deflection of the QRS complex is increased in leads that record left ventricular forces.
   - There is a deep S wave in leads $V_5$ and $V_6$.

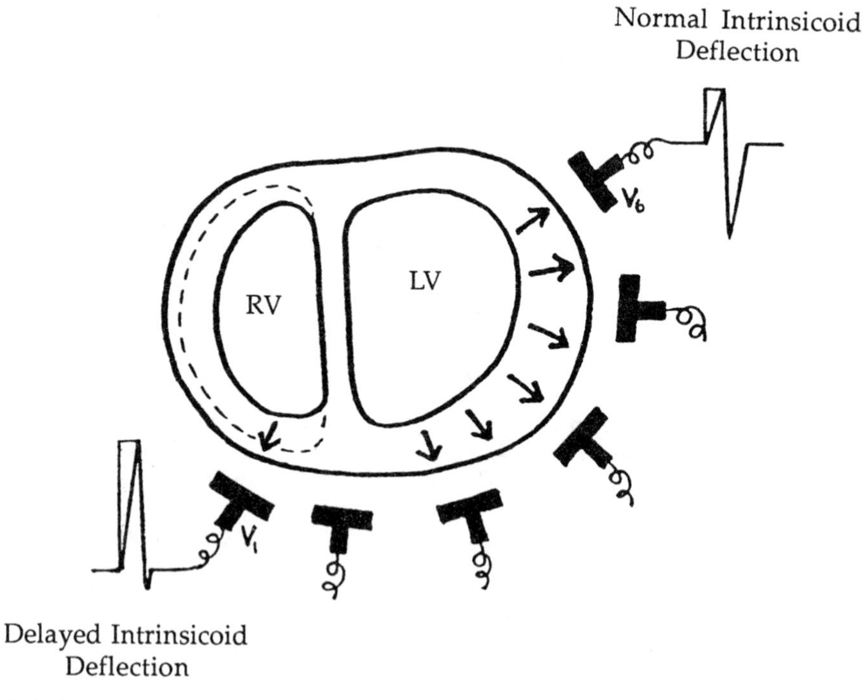

FIGURE 16-3. Right ventricular enlargement (hypertrophy). The onset of the intrinsicoid deflection is delayed in right chest lead $V_1$ because it takes longer than usual to depolarize the abnormally thick muscle (LV, left ventricle; RV, right ventricle).

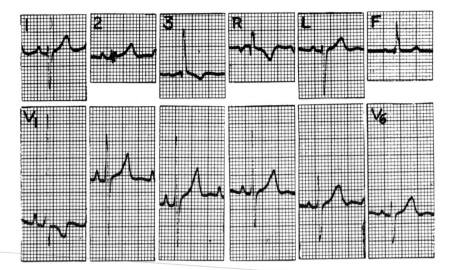

**FIGURE 16-4.** Right ventricular enlargement. The QRS complex in lead $V_1$ is predominantly positive with a much taller than expected R wave. The QRS complex in lead $V_6$ is predominantly negative with a deeper than expected S wave. Right axis deviation is present. (From Marriott, HJL: Practical Electrocardiography, ed 7. Williams & Wilkins, 1983, p 56, with permission.)

4. The onset of the intrinsicoid deflection is delayed beyond 0.02 second in right chest leads, but it remains normal in left chest leads (the time to onset of the intrinsicoid deflection reflects the time required to depolarize the ventricle from endocardium to epicardium; it is measured from the beginning of the QRS complex to the peak of the R wave; any increase in wall thickness will delay the onset of the intrinsicoid deflection in leads oriented over the hypertrophied chamber).

5. Incomplete RBBB may be present (rSR' in lead $V_1$).

6. QRS width may be slightly prolonged (greater than 0.10 second).

7. ST-T wave alterations: ST segment depression and T wave inversion in right chest leads $V_1$ and $V_2$ reflect secondary repolarization changes.

**Note:** *Right ventricular enlargement reverses normal R-wave progression in leads $V_1$ through $V_6$.*

## ECG CLUES TO LEFT VENTRICULAR ENLARGEMENT

Left ventricular enlargement exaggerates the normal R wave progression in leads $V_1$ through $V_6$. R waves get taller and S waves get deeper.

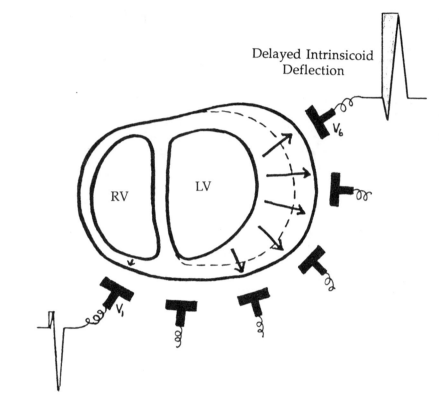

Delayed Intrinsicoid
Deflection

RV

LV

V₆

V₁

Normal Intrinsicoid
Deflection

**FIGURE 16-5.** Left ventricular enlargement (hypertrophy). The onset of the intrinsicoid deflection is delayed in left chest lead $V_6$ because it takes longer than usual to depolarize the abnormally thick muscle.

## ECG Criteria

1. Left axis deviation: the QRS axis is between $-30°$ and $-90°$ (the axis usually shifts because left ventricular muscle mass increases significantly).
2. The height (or voltage) of the QRS complex is increased in leads that record left ventricular forces (I, aVL, $V_5$, $V_6$); the depth of the QRS complex is increased in the right ventricular leads ($V_1$, $V_2$).*

---

*A simple method for determining LVH: Add the depth of the S wave in $V_1$ and the height of the R wave in $V_5$ or $V_6$ (whichever is greater); if the sum is greater than 35 mm, a diagnosis of left ventricular hypertrophy based on voltage criteria is achieved.

- The R wave is greater than 26 mm in leads $V_5$ or $V_6$ or greater than 11 mm in lead aVL.
- The height of the R wave in lead $V_5$ or $V_6$ plus the depth of the S wave in lead $V_1$ is greater than 35 mm.
- The S wave is deeper than expected in leads $V_1$ and $V_2$.

3. The onset of the intrinsicoid deflection is delayed beyond 0.04 second in left chest leads but remains normal in right chest leads.
4. QRS width is prolonged (beyond 0.09 second and up to 0.12 second).
5. ST-T wave alterations: ST segment depression and T wave inversion in left chest leads I, aVL, $V_4$, $V_5$, and $V_6$ reflect secondary repolarization changes.

---

**Note:** *Left ventricular enlargement causes increased QRS voltage in the chest leads; R waves grow taller and S waves deeper. Repolarization changes (in the ST segment and T wave) are also seen.*

---

Chamber enlargement is most often the result of chronic conditions that impose prolonged stress on the heart. Treatment options should focus on eradicating the underlying cause.

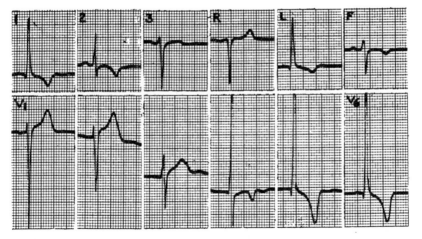

**FIGURE 16–6.** Left ventricular enlargement. The voltage of the QRS complexes is exaggerated, especially in the chest leads. Right-sided chest leads $V_1$ and $V_2$ are deeper than normal; left-sided chest leads $V_4$ to $V_6$ are taller than normal. Left axis deviation is present. (From Marriott, HJL: Practical Electrocardiography, ed 7. Williams & Wilkins, 1983, p 53, with permission.)

BOX 16–2 **Diagnosis of Left Ventricular Enlargement Based on Estes Criteria**

Left ventricular enlargement (commonly called left ventricular hypertrophy) may be diagnosed using a scoring system developed by Estes. At least five points are required to establish the diagnosis of LVH.

3 POINTS ~ VOLTAGE

3 POINTS ~ ST SEGMENT, T WAVE CHANGES

(EXCEPTION: 1 POINT IF PATIENT IS TAKING DIGITALIS)

3 POINTS ~ LEFT ATRIAL HYPERTROPHY

2 POINTS ~ LEFT AXIS DEVIATION

1 POINT ~ WIDENED QRS

1 POINT ~ DELAYED INTRINSICOID DEFLECTION

(Adapted from Romhilt, D and Estes, E: A point-score system for the ECG diagnoses of left ventricular hypertrophy. Am Heart J 75:752–758, 1968.)

# Chapter

# 17

# DISEASES AND DISORDERS

## ☐ PULMONARY EMBOLISM

A pulmonary embolus (PE) is a blood clot that embolizes to the lungs. When a clot (from peripheral veins, the right atrium, or the right ventricle) travels into the pulmonary circuit, it effectively blocks forward blood flow through a portion of the lung bed. If the embolus is large enough to block a major vessel (or multiple vessels), clinically significant signs and symptoms are likely to occur. High pressure builds up in the pulmonary circulation proximal to the blockage, and acute strain is placed on the right heart as it tries to pump blood past the obstruction. These acute mechanical changes may cause changes on the electrocardiogram, which can be useful in the differential diagnosis of pulmonary embolism.

*Note: Pulmonary embolus causes acute strain on the right heart (right atrium and right ventricle).*

ECG clues to acute pulmonary embolism may appear suddenly, and include:

1. An S wave in lead I, a Q wave in lead III, and an inverted T wave in lead III (the classic triad of ECG findings—$S_1Q_3T_3$)
2. Acute right axis deviation (due to strain on the right heart)
3. P pulmonale with tall, peaked P waves seen best in leads II, III, and aVF
4. New right bundle branch block (RBBB)
5. Sudden appearance of ST segment depression, T wave inversion, or Q waves in the inferior or anterior leads (simulates the ECG signs of myocardial ischemia or infarction)

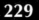

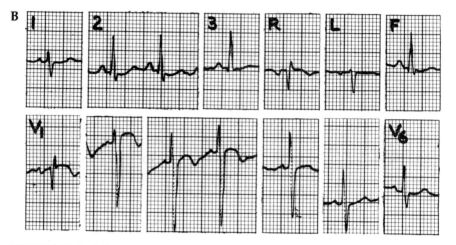

**FIGURE 17-1.** Pulmonary embolus. The classic combination $S_1Q_3T_3$ is present. There is slight right axis deviation. P-pulmonale is evident in the inferior leads; T wave inversion is present in chest leads $V_1$ to $V_4$. (From Marriott, HJL: Pearls & Pitfalls in Electrocardiography. Lea & Febiger, Philadelphia, 1990, p 131, with permission.)

Pulmonary embolus can be accompanied by a variety of supraventricular dysrhythmias, including sinus tachycardia, atrial flutter, atrial fibrillation, and paroxysmal supraventricular tachycardia.

Inasmuch as the clinical picture changes rapidly during acute PE, the ECG changes quickly as well. Serial ECGs are important in order accurately to diagnose an acute PE.

Treatment options include oxygen, bed rest, heparin therapy, and thrombolytic therapy.

# ◻ PERICARDITIS

Pericarditis represents diffuse inflammation of the pericardial lining surrounding the heart. Although it may appear as a complication of acute myocardial infarction, pericarditis is also associated with a host of pathologies, many of which may be noncardiac in origin.

The primary ECG clue to the presence of pericarditis is *widespread ST segment elevation* appearing in every lead except aVR (where ST segment depression may be seen). Other clues include:

1. The ST segment elevation is concave upward.
2. PR segment depression may be present and is best seen in lead I.
3. Pericarditis does not produce pathologic Q waves.
4. As pericarditis resolves, the elevated ST segments return to normal, but the T waves may invert or become biphasic and remain that way for weeks or months.

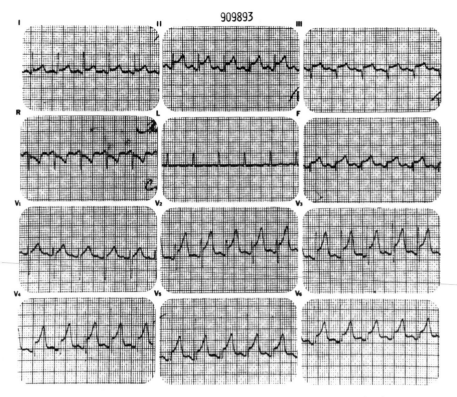

**909893**

**FIGURE 17-2.** Pericarditis. ST segment elevation is visible in every lead except aVR. Also note sinus tachycardia at a rate of 130 bpm. (From Andreoli, TE, Carpenter, CCJ, Plum, F, and Smith, LH: Cecil Essentials of Medicine. WB Saunders, Philadelphia, 1986, p 105, with permission.)

---

*Note: Pericarditis causes widespread ST segment elevation.*

---

Pericarditis may be accompanied by acute clinical signs and symptoms, including:

1. Sharp chest pain that increases with inspiration
2. Fever
3. Tachycardia
4. Pericardial friction rub (upon auscultation of the heart, a friction rub sounds like two pieces of sandpaper rubbing together); possibly transient
5. Pericardial effusion (fluid surrounding the heart), manifested on the ECG by low-voltage QRS complexes

**CLINICAL TIP**

Both pericarditis (widespread inflammation) and acute myocardial infarction (localized tissue damage) are accompanied by chest pain and ECG changes, so the clinical history and physical examination, as well as ECG clues, must be considered before making a diagnosis. The symptoms of pericarditis can mimic those of acute myocardial infarction.

Pericarditis may be treated with anti-inflammatory drugs, including aspirin. Narcotic analgesics are usually required to blunt the intense pain that persists until pericardial inflammation subsides.

# ☐ VENTRICULAR ANEURYSM

Ventricular aneurysm is an outpouching of the ventricular wall that results from stretching of previously infarcted heart muscle. An aneurysm is composed primarily of scar tissue and develops over a period of weeks to months after an acute myocardial infarction.

**Note:** *Ventricular aneurysm is an outpouching of the ventricular wall.*

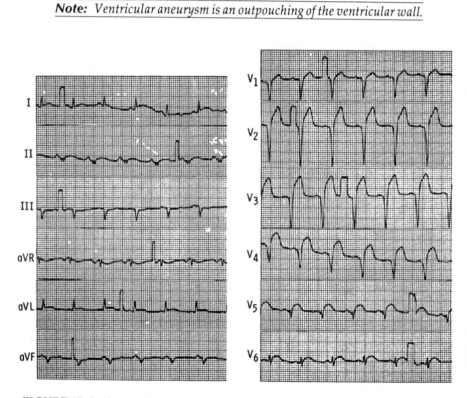

**FIGURE 17-3.** Ventricular aneurysm. Persistent ST segment elevation (especially in the chest leads) is demonstrated in a patient with a history of anterior and diaphragmatic wall myocardial infarction. (From Chung, EK: Electrocardiography: Practical Applications with Vectorial Principles, ed 3. Appleton & Lange, Norwalk, CT, 1985, p 689, with permission.)

The ECG hallmark of ventricular aneurysm is *persistent ST segment elevation.* Other clues:

1. ST segment elevation continues in the same leads in which it was observed during the acute event.
2. ST segment elevation may persist for years (compare recent ECGs with old tracings).
3. Persistent ST segment elevation may be associated with metastatic tumor of the ventricle (rare).

> **Note:** *Ventricular aneurysm causes persistent ST segment elevation.*

Ventricular aneurysm can be associated with two potentially dangerous clinical problems. First, a **mural thrombus** may form in the aneurysm and rarely embolize. Second, the area adjacent to the ventricular aneurysm may become a focus for serious **ventricular dysrhythmias.** Therapy includes conventional antidysrhythmic drug therapy, ablation procedures, surgical interventions, or insertion of an implantable cardioverter defibrillator (ICD).

> **Note:** *Ventricular aneurysm may be associated with mural thrombi and ventricular dysrhythmias.*

# ☐ WOLFF-PARKINSON-WHITE SYNDROME

The Wolff-Parkinson-White (WPW) syndrome represents a form of ventricular preexcitation in which the ventricles are depolarized using both a congenital accessory bypass tract and normal atrioventricular (AV) conduction pathways.

> **Note:** *WPW is a form of ventricular preexcitation.*

The accessory bypass tract (called the bundle of Kent) links either the left atrium and ventricle (type A) or the right atrium and ventricle (type B). The AV node is bypassed completely, so an impulse conducted along the accessory tract enters the ventricles early (preexcitation), causing abnormal ventricular depolarization. Because the impulse does not encounter normal delay at the AV node, the PR interval is abnormally short. Rapid conduction into the ventricles along the bypass tract causes slurring of the initial QRS deflection (called a delta wave) and widening of the QRS complex. Conduction also proceeds normally through the AV node, so the QRS complex represents fusion of normal and abnormal depolarization forces.

> **Note:** *In WPW, the impulse enters the ventricles early because it is conducted along the bundle of Kent, bypassing the AV node.*

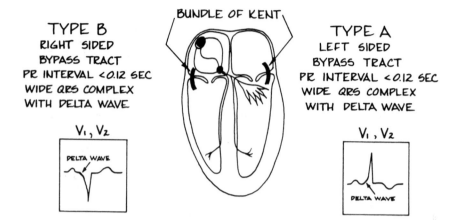

TYPE B
RIGHT SIDED
BYPASS TRACT
PR INTERVAL <0.12 SEC
WIDE QRS COMPLEX
WITH DELTA WAVE

$V_1, V_2$

DELTA WAVE

BUNDLE OF KENT

TYPE A
LEFT SIDED
BYPASS TRACT
PR INTERVAL <0.12 SEC
WIDE QRS COMPLEX
WITH DELTA WAVE

$V_1, V_2$

DELTA WAVE

**FIGURE 17–4.** Preexcitation of the ventricles using an accessory bypass tract. The Bundle of Kent links the atrium with the ventricle. It allows the impulse to enter the ventricles rapidly, bypassing normal delay at the AV node. The resulting PR interval is abnormally short, and the initial deflection of the QRS complex is slurred (called a "delta wave"). (From Lipman, BC and Lipman, BS: ECG Pocket Guide. Year Book Medical Publishers, 1987, p 136, with permission.)

ECG clues to WPW include:

1. Short PR interval (less than 0.12 second)
2. Slurring of the initial QRS deflection (delta wave)
   - Type A associated with positive QRS complex in lead $V_1$
   - Type B associated with negative QRS complex in lead $V_1$
3. Wide QRS

**Note:** *The hallmark of WPW is the presence of a delta wave.*

# ☐ CHRONIC OBSTRUCTIVE PULMONARY DISEASE

Chronic obstructive pulmonary disease (COPD) is associated with a host of clinical problems including increased airways resistance, alveolar and pulmonary capillary destruction, air trapping, chronic hypoxemia, and increased work of breathing. In an attempt to improve oxygenation of the blood, pulmonary vessels adjacent to underventilated alveoli tend to constrict, increasing both pulmonary vascular resistance and the work of the right heart.

**Note:** *COPD imposes chronic strain on the right heart.*

A

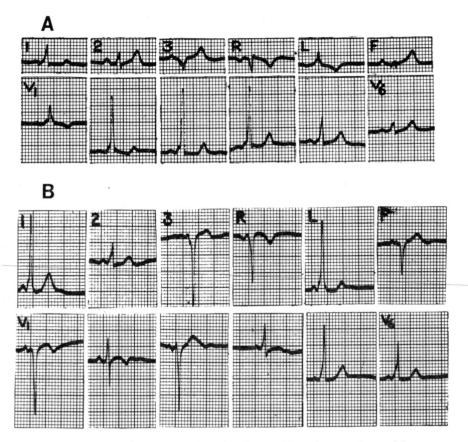

B

**FIGURE 17-5.** Wolff-Parkinson-White Syndrome. Note the prominent delta wave visible in multiple leads. The QRS complex is wide because the initial QRS deflection is slurred. (*A*) WPW, type A. The QRS complex is positive in lead $V_1$. (*B*) WPW, type B. The QRS complex is negative in lead $V_1$. (From Marriott, HJL: Practical Electrocardiography, ed 7. Williams & Wilkins, Baltimore, 1983, p 259, with permission.)

ECG clues associated with COPD include:

1. P pulmonale (reflects right atrial abnormality; see p 220)
2. Increased R wave voltage in leads $V_1$ and $V_2$ (reflects right ventricular enlargement)
3. Right axis deviation usually between $+90°$ and $+180°$ (reflects right ventricular dilatation)
4. Low-voltage QRS complexes (less than 5 mm) in the limb leads (air trapping causes hyperinflation of the lungs and increases the distance between the surface ECG electrode and the heart)

BOX 17–1 **Other Forms of Preexcitation**

Other forms of ventricular preexcitation include Lown-Ganong-Levine (LGL) syndrome and the Mahaim bypass tract syndrome; LGL syndrome is associated with the James bypass tract. Like WPW, these syndromes use an accessory bypass tract that allows early depolarization of the ventricles, but neither syndrome produces a delta wave on the ECG.

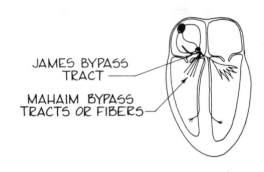

JAMES BYPASS TRACT ———

MAHAIM BYPASS TRACTS OR FIBERS—

The James Bypass Tract and the Mahaim Bypass Tracts are two other accessory pathways associated with ventricular preexcitation. (From Lipman, BC and Lipman, BS: ECG Pocket Guide. Year Book Medical Publishers, Chicago, 1987, p 137, with permission.)

5. Poor R wave progression (hyperinflated lungs may push down on the heart, causing leftward, or clockwise, rotation of the heart); poor R wave progression may simulate anterior myocardial infarction
6. Supraventricular dysrhythmias, including atrial premature complexes (APCs), atrial flutter, atrial fibrillation, paroxysmal atrial tachycardia, and multifocal atrial tachycardia

*Note:* ECG findings of right atrial and right ventricular enlargement are seen with COPD.

*Note:* Multifocal atrial tachycardia (MAT) is commonly associated with severe COPD or exacerbation of lung disease.

# ☐ CEREBROVASCULAR ACCIDENT

Cerebrovascular accident (CVA) may be accompanied by ECG changes probably reflecting changes in the autonomic nervous system during the acute event. These changes primarily affect repolarization and usually resolve over time.

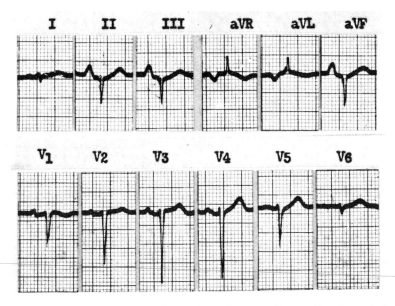

**FIGURE 17-6.** COPD = chronic obstructive pulmonary disease. P-pulmonale is evident in the leads II, III, and aVF. Note the poor R wave progression, low voltage QRS complexes in the limb leads, and right axis deviation. (From Lipman, BC and Lipman, BS: ECG Pocket Guide. Year Book Medical Publishers, Chicago, 1987, p 134, with permission.)

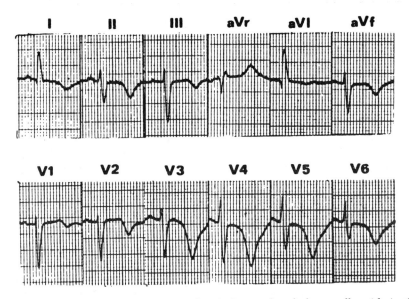

**FIGURE 17-7.** CVA. The T waves are deeply inverted and abnormally wide in the chest leads. The QT interval is prolonged. (From Lipman, BC and Lipman, BS: ECG Pocket Guide. Year Book Medical Publishers, Chicago, 1987, p 127, with permission.) CVA = cerebrovascular accident

> *Note: CVA may cause repolarization changes on the ECG.*

ECG changes associated with CVA are quite variable, and may include:

1. Tall and peaked or deeply inverted T waves
2. Abnormally wide T waves
3. Prolonged QT interval
4. Prominent u waves
5. Q waves simulating myocardial infarction

# ☐ HYPOTHERMIA

Hypothermia (low core body temperature) may be caused by environmental exposure and is aggravated by taking vasodilating drugs and drinking alcohol. Hypothermia may also be medically induced in conjunction with cardiac surgery or other procedures.

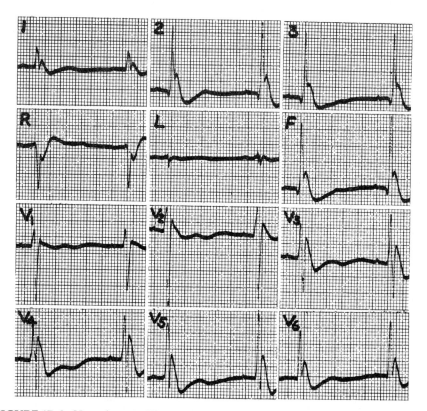

**FIGURE 17–8.** Hypothermia. The Osborn wave (or J wave) is easily visible, especially in the chest leads. (From Marriott, HJL: Practical Electrocardiography, ed 7. Williams & Wilkins, Baltimore, 1983, p 466, with permission.)

Prolonged exposure to critically low temperatures will profoundly depress both electrical and mechanical activity in the heart. Characteristic ECG changes are observed as core body temperature drops. ECG changes associated with hypothermia are variable and include:

1. Sinus bradycardia (core temperature 35° to 37°C)
2. Prolongation of the PR interval (core temperature 30° to 35°C)
3. Widening of the QRS complex (core temperature 30° to 35°C)
4. Lengthening of the ST segment and QT interval (core temperature 30° to 35°C)
5. Osborn wave (also called a J wave) in the terminal QRS complex (core temperature less than 30°C)
6. Ventricular dysrhythmias (core temperature less than 30°C)

**Note:** *The Osborn wave (J wave) is characteristic of hypothermia when core body temperature falls to 30°C.*

When core body temperature is critically low, the patient may appear clinically dead because of profound vital function depression. The immediate goal of therapy is to rewarm core blood as rapidly as possible. Caution should be exercised to minimize any adverse effects (e.g., life-threatening ventricular dysrhythmias) associated with rapid rewarming of the body.

# Chapter

# 18

# STRESS TESTING AND HOLTER MONITORING

## ☐ STRESS TESTING

Stress testing is a noninvasive method for evaluation of heart disease. The patient usually exercises on a treadmill or bicycle ergometer and is continuously monitored. Normal exercise-related electrocardiogram (ECG) changes include an increase in the heart rate, shorter PR and QT intervals, a decrease in the height of the R wave, and mild depression of the J point with upsloping of the ST segment. Abnormal ECG changes may be observed in the presence of heart disease and other conditions (such as hypertension or left ventricular enlargement) or as a normal variant.

*Note:* *Stress testing is a noninvasive method to evaluate heart disease.*

The sensitivity and specificity of stress testing can be enhanced with the addition of thallium, technetium, and positron emission tomography (PET) imaging as well as with echocardiography.

Newer methods of stressing the heart without exercising are also being used. These include administration of intravenous dipyridamole, adenosine, dobutamine, and other agents that are under investigation. As with conventional exercise stress testing, ECG monitoring is performed during these procedures. Thallium, technetium, echocardiography, and PET scanning are used routinely with these IV agents.

*Note:* *Administration of dipyridamole, adenosine, and other agents are alternatives to exercise stress testing for those who cannot exercise.*

ECG analysis during exercise testing focuses on the J point and ST segment as well as on the presence of dysrhythmias, especially those of ventricular origin. Criteria for diagnosis of a positive stress test include:

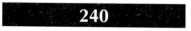

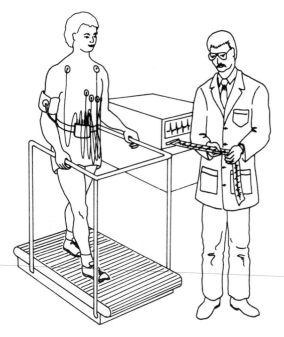

**FIGURE 18–1.** Exercise treadmill. The ECG and blood pressure are continuously monitored while the patient walks in place on a treadmill. The slope and speed of the treadmill are gradually increased during the test. (From Lipman, BC and Lipman, BS: ECG Pocket Guide. Year Book Medical Publishers, Chicago, 1987, p 146, with permission.)

1. **Depression of the J point and ST segment** (horizontal depression or downsloping of the ST segment by 1 mm or more below the baseline is abnormal). The severity of heart disease can be gauged by the depth of ST segment depression, the rapidity with which it occurs after exercise begins, and the total length of time that it persists following exercise.
2. **Elevation of the J point and ST segment** by 1 mm or more above the baseline (in the absence of preexisting ST segment elevation).
3. The height of the R wave is increased.
4. The u waves are inverted.

> **Note:** *A positive stress test causes either depression or elevation of the J point and ST segment.*

It is important to note that *false-positive* ECG changes during stress testing may occur in a variety of situations, including:

1. Treatment with digitalis
2. Hypokalemia
3. Preexisting ST segment abnormalities

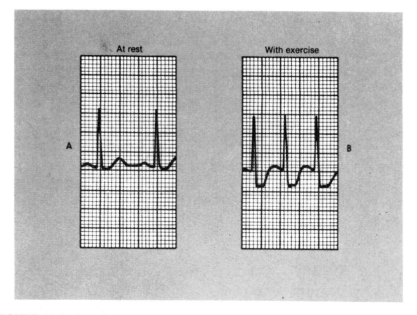

**FIGURE 18–2.** A positive exercise stress test. ST segment depression appears during exercise in the ECG example on the right. (From Canobbio, MM: Cardiovascular Disorders. CV Mosby, St. Louis, 1990, p 81, with permission.)

4. Underlying ventricular hypertrophy
5. Baseline left bundle branch block (LBBB)
6. Preexisting WPW syndrome
7. Mitral valve prolapse
8. In female patients (for unknown reasons)

**Note:** *False-positive stress test results occur in a variety of situations.*

# ☐ HOLTER MONITORING

Holter monitoring is a method of continuously recording cardiac rhythms over a specified period of time. The test can be conducted on an outpatient basis and is used to detect dysrhythmias as well as episodes of ischemia or coronary artery spasm.

**Note:** *Holter monitoring is used to evaluate dysrhythmias and episodes of ischemia or coronary artery spasm.*

The patient wears monitoring electrodes attached to a portable device that records the cardiac rhythm continuously over a period of 12, 24, or 48 hours. The patient conducts normal activities of daily living while the test is in progress and is asked to record significant events and any associated symptoms in

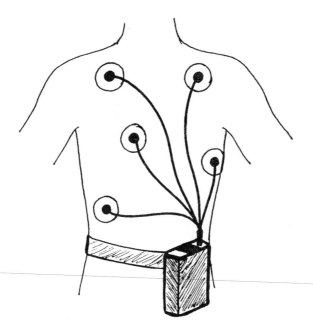

**FIGURE 18-3.** Holter monitoring. Electrodes placed on the body surface record the ECG continously over a period of hours to days.

a diary (including the time). At the completion of the test, the stored rhythm is scanned to detect dysrhythmias, heart blocks, or ST segment changes. Events noted in the diary (including associated symptoms) are correlated with the cardiac rhythms recorded on the Holter tracing at that time. One practical drawback to Holter monitoring is the variable accuracy of entries in the patient's diary.

> **Note:** *The ECG is recorded continuously while a diary of activities and their associated symptoms is kept by the patient. Accuracy of the patient diary is very important in the evaluation of Holter data.*

It is important to consider the following with respect to Holter monitoring:

1. Patients with impaired eyesight may have difficulty documenting in the diary.
2. Patients with impaired memory (often the elderly) may forget to document in the diary.

Clearly, pretest instruction must emphasize the importance of documenting all significant activities and their associated symptoms.

# Chapter

# 19

# CARDIAC TRANSPLANTATION

Cardiac transplantation is performed when conventional therapy fails to improve the clinical outlook for the patient with end-stage heart disease. The most common procedure is called orthotopic heart transplantation; the recipient's heart is excised and replaced with a donor heart. The heterotopic transplant piggybacks the donor's heart onto the recipient's heart, but this procedure is currently performed in relatively few centers.

*Note: Orthotopic transplantation involves nearly complete removal of the recipient's heart and replacement with a donor heart.*

In orthotopic transplantation, the native atrial cuffs are retained (to make suturing easier), but the ventricles are completely removed. Because the recipient's sinoatrial (SA) node is retained, native P waves may be observed on the electrocardiogram, but the native sinus impulses cannot cross the suture line and are not responsible for depolarizing the donor atria. Instead, the donor SA node takes over as the dominant pacemaker for the transplanted heart. The ECG reveals independent P waves (remnant P waves from the native SA node) that march through the dominant rhythm but are unrelated to it. Remnant P waves usually disappear over time.

*Note: Remnant P waves may be seen marching through the underlying donor cardiac rhythm.*

The transplanted heart does not adjust its rate the way a normal heart does. It cannot respond to catecholamines (epinephrine and norepinephrine) released from nerve endings because all nerves are cut during the procedure. Instead, the transplanted heart relies on blood-borne catecholamines to control heart rate. It is important to remember that the transplanted heart will *not* respond to atropine (a parasympathetic blocking agent). Symptomatic bradycardia may be treated with a beta agonist drug such as isoproterenol.

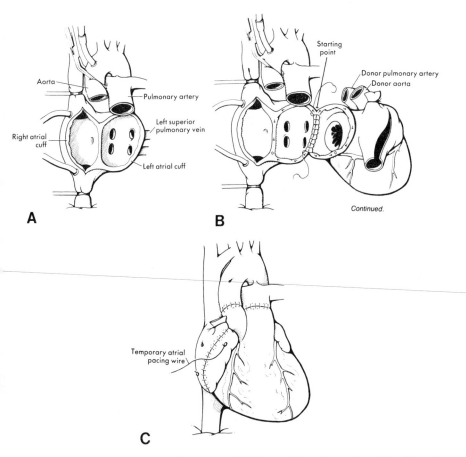

**FIGURE 19–1.** Orthotopic transplantation. (*A*) The recipient (native) atrial cuffs and great vessels after cardioectomy. (*B*) The donor atrial cuffs are sutured to the native cuffs; the beginning of the left atrial suture line is shown here. (*C*) The transplant is complete. (From Zschoche, DA: Mosby's Comprehensive Review of Critical Care, ed 3. CV Mosby, 1986, pp 483, 484, with permission.)

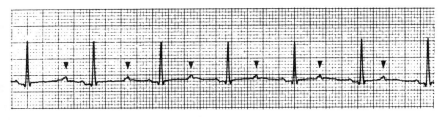

**FIGURE 19–2.** Remnant P waves. The recipient's native SA node (retained in the right atrial cuff) continues to generate P waves (*arrows*) that are unrelated to the donor P waves. Note the difference in the shape of the donor and recipient P waves. (From Smith, SL: Tissue and Organ Transplantation: Implications for Professional Nursing Practice. Mosby Year Book, St. Louis, 1990, p 224, with permission.)

Rejection is a feared but often treatable complication of transplantation. The diagnosis is based on analysis of biopsied cardiac tissue, cardiac ultrasound, and ECG findings. ECG clues may include:

1. Low-voltage QRS complexes
2. Prolonged PR interval
3. Right axis deviation
4. Right bundle branch block (RBBB)
5. Supraventricular dysrhythmias (e.g., atrial premature complexes [APCs], atrial tachycardia with block, atrial fibrillation, junctional escape rhythm)
6. Ventricular dysrhythmias (primarily ventricular premature complexes [VPCs])

When the rejection episode resolves, the ECG will usually normalize.

# Chapter

# 20

# DRUGS AND ELECTROLYTES

## ☐ DRUG EFFECTS

### DIGITALIS

Digitalis glycosides are given to enhance myocardial performance in situations of chronic heart failure as well as to control many supraventricular dysrhythmias. Normal serum levels of digoxin may produce subtle alterations in the electrocardiogram called the digitalis effect or "dig. effect." Toxic levels are associated with potentially life-threatening dysrhythmias, heart blocks, and other clinically significant side effects.

ECG manifestations of the "dig. effect" include:

1. Depressed ST segments in leads where the main QRS deflection is positive (e.g., in the inferior and lateral leads); the ST segments gradually slope downward and look "scooped out"
2. Elevated ST segments in leads where the main QRS deflection is negative (e.g., lead $V_1$)
3. Flattened or inverted T waves
4. Shortened QT interval
5. Prolongation of the PR interval compared with a pretreatment baseline; the PR interval often lengthens by 0.04 to 0.08 second (or more)

*Note:* *"Dig. effect" is associated with alterations in the ST segment and PR interval.*

No treatment is usually required, but continued observation is recommended to detect the onset of new dysrhythmias, heart block, or significant clinical symptoms.

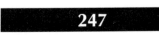

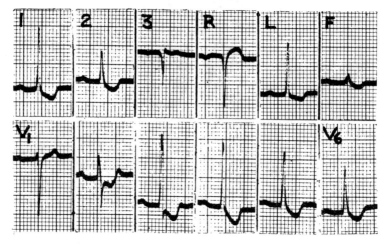

**FIGURE 20-1.** "Dig." effect. The ST segments are depressed, with a "scooped out" look in several leads. (From Marriott, HJL: Practical Electrocardiography, ed 7. Williams & Wilkins, Baltimore, 1983, p 425, with permission.)

ECG manifestations of digitalis toxicity include:

1. The same ST segment and T wave changes noted with the "dig. effect"
2. *Significant* prolongation of the PR interval
3. Supraventricular dysrhythmias (e.g., extreme sinus bradycardia, atrial premature complexes [APCs], sinoatrial [SA] block, junctional premature complexes [JPCs], junctional escape rhythm, accelerated junctional rhythm, junctional tachycardia, atrial tachycardia with AV block)
4. Ventricular dysrhythmias (e.g., ventricular premature complexes [VPCs], ventricular bigeminy, ventricular tachycardia [VT], and ventricular fibrillation [VF]); bidirectional VT (alternating polarity of the QRS complex) is associated with a poor prognosis
5. Atrioventricular (AV) block (e.g., atrial tachycardia with AV block; second-degree AV block, type I; and third-degree AV block)

---
**Note:** *Digitalis toxicity is associated with varying degrees of AV block and dangerous ventricular dysrhythmias.*

---

Digitalis preparations have a narrow therapeutic range, so maintaining the desirable serum level of the drug is difficult, even under ideal conditions. Antidysrhythmic agents such as quinidine and amiodarone, as well as the calcium channel blocker verapamil, are known to increase the serum digoxin level. Hypokalemia, a common side effect of diuretic therapy, also potentiates the toxic effects of digitalis.

**CLINICAL TIP**
Many drugs can increase the serum digoxin level. Hypokalemia potentiates digitalis toxicity.

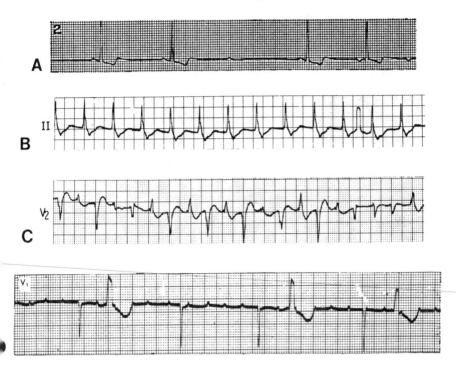

**FIGURE 20-2.** Digitalis toxicity. A wide variety of dysrhythmias and heart blocks may accompany digitalis toxicity. (*A*) The initial portion of this rhythm is sinus bradycardia. Toward the end of the strip an ectopic junctional pacemaker takes over; note the inverted P wave preceding the last QRS complex. (Marriott, HJL: Practical Electrocardiography, ed 7. Williams & Wilkins, Baltimore, 1983, p 432, with permission.) (*B*) Junctional tachycardia at approximately 100 bpm. Note the inverted P wave in the terminal portion of the QRS complex. (From Chung, EK: Electrocardiography: Practical Applications with Vectorial Principles, ed 3. Appleton & Lange, Norwalk, CT, 1985, p 517, with permission.) (*C*) Atrial fibrillation with bidirectional ventricular tachycardia. There is alternating polarity of the QRS complexes. Bidirectional VT is associated with advanced digitalis toxicity and a poor prognosis. (From Chung, EK: Electrocardiography: Practical Applications with Vectorial Principles, ed 3. Appleton & Lange, Norwalk, CT, 1985, p 514, with permission.) (*D*) Atrial tachycardia with 4:1 AV block and ventricular ectopic complexes. (From Marriott, HJL and Conover, MB: Advanced Concepts in Arrhythmias, ed 2. CV Mosby Company, St. Louis, 1989, p 66, with permission.)

Treatment of digitalis toxicity includes:

1. Withholding further digoxin
2. Potassium replacement therapy (carefully, avoid hyperkalemia)
3. Digoxin antibody fragments (digoxin immune Fab)
4. Temporary pacing
5. Diphenylhydantoin (for treatment of digitalis-induced ventricular dysrhythmias)

## ANTIDYSRHYTHMIC DRUGS

Antidysrhythmic agents are generally classified according to their effects on the action potential. The widely used Vaughan Williams* system, for example, describes four classes of cardiac drugs and places most antidysrhythmic drugs into class I. Drugs in this class exert their primary effects on the fast sodium channel, altering depolarization and, to some extent, repolarization. Subgroups IA, IB, and IC distinguish class I drugs even further.

Drugs found in the other three Vaughan Williams classes will not be discussed in detail. Class II drugs are beta blockers; class III drugs prolong repolarization (e.g., bretylium, amiodarone, and others); and class IV drugs are calcium channel blockers.

### Class IA Drugs

Class IA drugs, which include quinidine, procainamide, and disopyramide, are given to treat both supraventricular and ventricular dysrhythmias. Despite their proven efficacy, these drugs can be proarrhythmic and can be associated with many side effects.

ECG effects associated with the use of class IA drugs are:

1. Prolonged QT interval (may lead to torsade de pointes)
2. Widening of the QRS complex (associated with toxic drug levels)
3. ST segment depression
4. T wave inversion
5. u wave prominence

Clinical side effects include:

1. Gastrointestinal disturbances, including diarrhea (common with quinidine)

---

*Vaughan Williams, EM. A classification of antiarrhythmic actions reassessed after a decade of new drugs. J Clin Pharmacol 24:129–147, 1984.

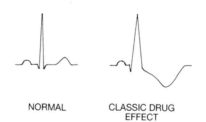

NORMAL          CLASSIC DRUG
                  EFFECT

FIGURE 20–3. ECG effects of class IA drugs. Class IA drugs are associated with prolongation of the QT interval, ST segment depression, and widening of the QRS complex.

2. Lupuslike syndrome (associated with procainamide)
3. Hypotension
4. Dry mouth and urinary retention (associated with disopyramide)
5. Syncope (possibly related to drug-induced torsade de pointes and other potential proarrhythmias such as refractory VT)
6. Increased serum digoxin level (associated with quinidine)

## Class IB Drugs

Class IB drugs include lidocaine, tocainide, mexiletine, and phenytoin. They are all given to treat ventricular dysrhythmias, but phenytoin may be used when the disturbances are caused by digitalis. The prototype IB drug is lidocaine. Tocainide and mexiletine are oral agents that are similar to lidocaine. Drugs in this group may be associated with many side effects.

The primary ECG effect associated with the use of class IB drugs is a *shortened QT interval.* Clinical side effects include:

1. Slurred speech, headache, tremors, paresthesias, seizures
2. Ataxia
3. Gingival hyperplasia (phenytoin)
4. Nausea (mexiletine, tocainide)

## Class IC Drugs

Class IC drugs, including flecainide, encainide, and propafenone, may be used to treat both supraventricular and ventricular dysrhythmias. These drugs can also be proarrhythmic, and their indications are being evaluated at this time.

ECG effects associated with the use of class IC drugs are:

1. Prolongation of the PR interval
2. Prolongation of the QRS complex and QT interval
3. Serious and refractory ventricular dysrhythmias

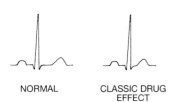

NORMAL          CLASSIC DRUG
                EFFECT

**FIGURE 20-4.** ECG effects of class IB drugs. Class IB drugs are associated with shortening of the QT interval.

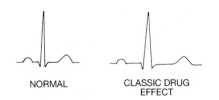

NORMAL                CLASSIC DRUG
                          EFFECT

**FIGURE 20-5.** ECG effects of class IC drugs. Class IC drugs are associated with prolongation of the PR and QT intervals and widening of the QRS complex.

Clinical side effects include:

1. Gastrointestinal upset
2. Dysgeusia
3. Blurred vision
4. Dizziness
5. Vertigo

# ☐ ELECTROLYTE ABNORMALITIES

## HYPOKALEMIA

Hypokalemia refers to a serum potassium ($K^+$) level less than 3.5 mEq/liter.

> **Note:** Hypokalemia = Serum $K^+$ < 3.5 mEq/liter.

### Etiology

1. Alkalosis ($K^+$ decreases approximately 0.6 mEq/liter for each 0.1 unit increase in pH)
2. Renal tubular acidosis
3. Insulin effect
4. Hyperaldosteronism (e.g., Conn's syndrome)
5. Excessive licorice ingestion (causes increased aldosteronelike effect)
6. Diuretics
7. Vomiting or nasogastric suction
8. Diarrhea
9. Decreased dietary intake, including crash dieting
10. Excessive diaphoresis
11. Burns
12. Hypomagnesemia

## ECG Clues

Hypokalemia prolongs repolarization; changes in the T and u waves provide the earliest clues to low serum potassium. ECG effects include:

1. Decreased amplitude (flattening) of the T wave
2. T wave inversion
3. Prominent u waves (best seen in leads $V_2$ to $V_4$)
4. T-u fusion (fusion of the T wave and u wave)
5. ST segment depression
6. Prominent P wave
7. Prolongation of the PR interval
8. Atrial and ventricular dysrhythmias (e.g., APCs, VPCs, VT, and VF)

*Note: Hypokalemia causes low-voltage T waves and prominent u waves.*

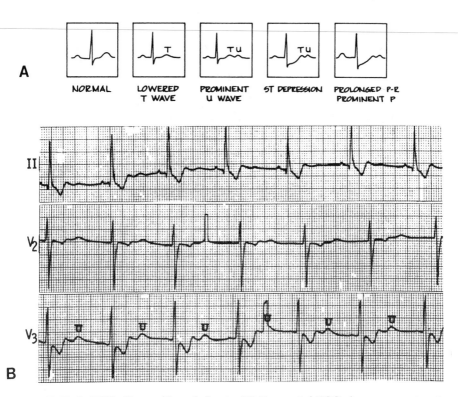

FIGURE 20-6. ECG effects of hypokalemia. (A) Sequential ECG changes associated with low serum potassium. (From Lipman, BC and Lipman, BS: ECG Pocket Guide. Year Book Medical Publishers, Chicago, 1987, p 124, with permission.) (B) Note the prominent u waves (best seen in lead $V_3$). (From Chung, EK: Electrocardiography: Practical Applications with Vectorial Principles, ed 3. Appleton & Lange, Norwalk, CT, 1985, p 530, with permission.)

## Treatment

1. Potassium replacement using oral or IV routes
2. Correction of the underlying cause

## Ongoing Care

1. Evaluate and manage the underlying cause of hypokalemia.
2. Monitor serum potassium levels periodically, especially when diuretics or digitalis preparations are given (hypokalemia potentiates the toxic effects of digitalis).
3. Give oral solutions in liquid (e.g., fruit juice) to minimize gastric irritation and enhance palatability.
4. Administer IV potassium through a large vessel; monitor complaints of burning at the IV site.
5. Do not give undiluted IV potassium (the usual admixture is 40 to 80 mEq of $K^+$ per liter)
6. Use caution when adding potassium to IV infusions; gently invert the container several times to mix the potassium with the solution (failure to do so may result in inadvertent bolusing of concentrated potassium).
7. Avoid rapid infusion of replacement potassium; avoid giving more than 10 mEq/hour through a peripheral vein or more than 20 mEq/hour through a central vein, except in extreme circumstances.
8. Connect the patient to a cardiac monitor during IV potassium replacement therapy, especially if the pretreatment serum potassium level is significantly low.
9. Monitor additional electrolyte abnormalities (e.g., hypomagnesemia).
10. Teach the patient about dietary sources of potassium (e.g., citrus fruits, bananas, tomatoes, peas).
11. Advise the patient to report signs and symptoms of hypokalemia such as muscle weakness and aching, abdominal distention, and constipation.

## HYPERKALEMIA

Hyperkalemia refers to a serum potassium ($K^+$) level greater than 5.1 mEq/liter.

*Note: Hyperkalemia = Serum $K^+$ > 5.1 mEq/liter.*

## Etiology

1. Renal failure
2. Adrenal insufficiency
3. Acidosis ($K^+$ increases approximately 0.6 mEq/liter for each 0.1 unit decrease in pH)

4. Trauma or ischemia (e.g., myocardial infarction, burns, hemolysis of red blood cells)
5. Potassium replacement therapy
6. Potassium-sparing drugs (such as spironolactone)
7. Drugs in a potassium-based carrier (such as potassium penicillin)

## ECG Clues
Hyperkalemia shortens repolarization; changes in the T wave provide the earliest clues to high serum potassium. ECG effects include:

1. Tall, symmetrically peaked T wave, best seen in leads $V_2$ to $V_4$
2. Widening of the QRS complex
3. QRS-T fusion (a sinusoidal waveform is observed when serum $K^+$ is critically elevated)
4. ST segment depression
5. Wide, flat P wave
6. Prolongation of the PR interval
7. Ventricular dysrhythmias (e.g., VT, ventricular flutter, VF, asystole)

*Note: Hyperkalemia causes tall, peaked T waves.*

## Treatment
1. Withholding of potassium replacement
2. IV calcium gluconate (to stabilize the myocardium)
3. Sodium bicarbonate
4. Glucose and insulin infusion
5. Potassium ion exchange resin
6. Dialysis
7. Diuretics (must not be a potassium-sparing agent)

## Ongoing Care
1. Evaluate and manage the underlying cause of hyperkalemia.
2. Prevent overcorrection during potassium replacement by monitoring serum potassium levels periodically; avoid hemolysis of the blood sample (causes a falsely elevated result).
3. Monitor blood gases for the appearance of acidosis.
4. Teach the patient about dietary sources of potassium (including unexpected sources, such as salt substitutes); excess dietary intake coupled with potassium-sparing drugs can promote hyperkalemia.

## HYPOMAGNESEMIA
Hypomagnesemia refers to a serum magnesium ($Mg^+$) level less than 1.5 mEq/liter.

*Note: Hypomagnesemia = Serum $Mg^+$ < 1.5 mEq/liter.*

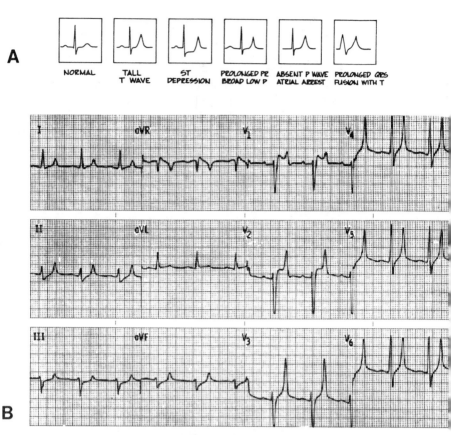

**FIGURE 20-7.** ECG effects of hyperkalemia. (*A*) Sequential ECG changes associated with high serum potassium. (From Lipman, BC and Lipman, BS: ECG Pocket Guide. Year Book Medical Publishers, Chicago, 1987, p 123, with permission.) (*B*) Moderate hyperkalemia is present in this example. The T waves are tall and peaked, the QRS complex is wider than normal, the ST segments are depressed in some leads, and the P waves are wide and flat in some leads. (From Chung, EK: Electrocardiography: Practical Applications with Vectorial Principles, ed 3. Appleton & Lange, Norwalk, CT, 1985, p 523, with permission.)

## Etiology
1. Diuretics
2. Gastrointestinal losses (vomiting, nasogastric suction, diarrhea, laxatives)
3. Inadequate dietary intake (e.g., associated with alcoholism)
4. Liver disease

## ECG Clues
ECG clues to hypomagnesemia are similar to those observed with hypokalemia. ECG effects include:

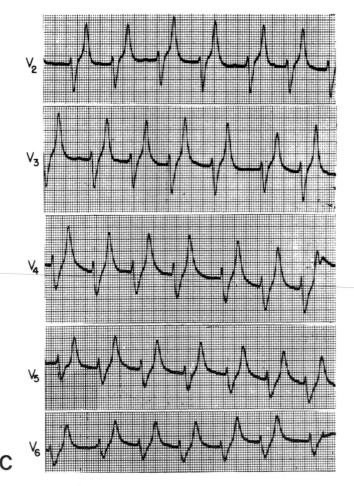

**FIGURE 20-7.** (*Continued*) (C) Significant hyperkalemia is present (8.8 mEq/per liter). The T waves are tall and peaked, the QRS complex is very wide, and the P waves are difficult to find. (From Lipman, BC and Lipman, BS: ECG Pocket Guide. Year Book Medical Publishers, Chicago, 1987, p 189, with permission.)

1. Prominent u waves
2. T wave flattening

## Treatment

1. Correct the underlying cause of hypomagnesemia.
2. Administer magnesium replacement therapy (oral or IV).

## Ongoing Care

1. Monitor serum magnesium levels periodically during replacement.
2. Monitor signs and symptoms of hypomagnesemia, including skeletal

and smooth muscle irritability (e.g., muscle cramping and spasms), confusion, disorientation, and seizures.

## HYPERMAGNESEMIA

Hypermagnesemia refers to a serum magnesium ($Mg^+$) level greater than 2.5 mEq/liter.

**Note:** *Hypermagnesemia = Serum $Mg^+ > 2.5$ mEq/liter.*

### Etiology
1. Renal failure
2. Hypothyroidism
3. Dehydration
4. Magnesium-containing antacids
5. Excess magnesium replacement

### ECG Clues
ECG clues to hypermagnesemia are similar to those observed with hyperkalemia. ECG effects include:

1. Tall, peaked T waves
2. Widening of the QRS complex

### Treatment
1. Correct the underlying cause of hypermagnesemia.
2. Stop magnesium replacement therapy.

### Ongoing Care
1. Monitor serum magnesium levels periodically during replacement; avoid hemolysis of the blood sample (causes a falsely elevated result).
2. Monitor signs of hypermagnesemia, including central nervous system depression, loss of deep tendon reflexes, bradycardia, and hypotension.

## HYPOCALCEMIA

Hypocalcemia refers to total **ionized** calcium ($CA^{++}$) level less than 4.5 mEq/liter. It is ionized calcium (not protein-bound calcium) that exerts an effect on the ECG.

**Note:** *Hypocalcemia = Ionized $Ca^{++} < 4.5$ mEq/liter.*

### Etiology
1. Alkalosis
2. Hypoparathyroidism

3. Disorders of vitamin D metabolism
4. Renal failure
5. Acute pancreatitis
6. Transfusions of stored blood (the preservative citrate binds with ionized calcium)
7. Malabsorption

## ECG Clues
1. Lengthening of the ST segment
2. Lengthening of the QT interval (primarily from the lengthened ST segment)
3. Atrial and ventricular dysrhythmias, including torsade de pointes (especially when accompanied by hypomagnesemia)

## Treatment
1. Correction of the underlying cause of hypocalcemia
2. Calcium replacement therapy
3. Vitamin D

## Ongoing Care
1. Evaluate and treat the underlying cause of hypocalcemia.
2. Monitor serum calcium levels periodically during calcium administration.
3. Avoid overzealous calcium replacement.
4. Use caution if calcium is given with digitalis glycosides (their effects are synergistic).
5. Do not give calcium preparations with sodium bicarbonate (they will precipitate).
6. Give IV calcium slowly; calcium chloride has a higher calcium content than calcium gluconate, but the latter is less irritating to blood vessels.

## HYPERCALCEMIA

Hypercalcemia refers to a total **ionized** calcium ($Ca^{++}$) level greater than 5.3 mEq/liter.

*Note: Hypercalcemia = Ionized $Ca^{++}$ > 5.3 mEq/liter.*

## Etiology
1. Hyperparathyroidism, especially in the presence of renal failure
2. Metastatic cancers
3. Immobility
4. Certain lung diseases such as sarcoidosis
5. Vitamin D intoxication

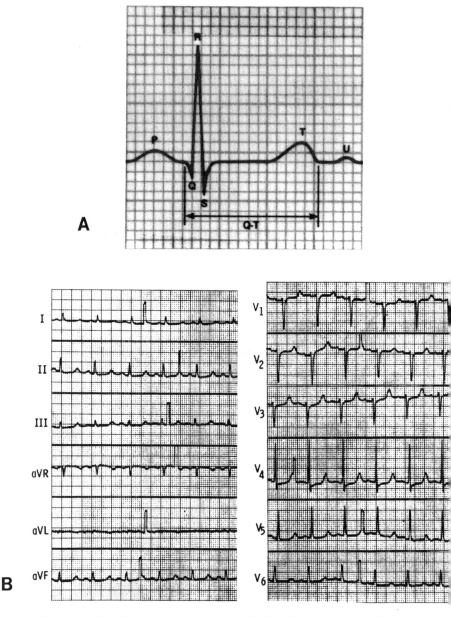

**FIGURE 20-8.** ECG effects of hypocalcemia. (*A*) The ST segment and QT interval lengthen with low levels of serum calcium. (From Dolan, JT: Critical Care Nursing: Clinical Management Through the Nursing Process. FA Davis, Philadelphia, 1991, p 827, with permission.) (*B*) Note the prolonged ST segment and QT interval consistent with hypocalcemia. (From Chung, EK: Electrocardiography: Practical Applications with Vectorial Principles, ed 3. Appleton & Lange, Norwalk, CT, 1985, p 533, with permission.)

6. Adrenal insufficiency
7. Milk-alkali syndrome

## ECG Clues
1. Shortening of the ST segment
2. Shortening of the QT interval
3. The end of the QRS indistinguishable from the beginning of the T wave
4. J wave (a small notch at the end of the QRS complex also observed in hypothermia); also called an Osborn wave
5. Atrial and ventricular dysrhythmias (especially if the patient is taking digoxin)

## Treatment
1. Hydration
2. Diuretics (to promote $Ca^{++}$ elimination by the kidneys)
3. Phosphate administration
4. Sodium bicarbonate (to bind excess calcium)
5. Steroids

## Ongoing Care
1. Evaluate and treat the underlying cause.
2. Monitor serum calcium levels periodically during replacement.

## ❑ UNIT KEY POINTS

- Chamber dilatation cannot be differentiated from chamber hypertrophy using the ECG alone.
- Atrial chamber enlargement, also called atrial abnormality, causes changes in the P wave.
- Tall, peaked P waves (P pulmonale) are associated with right atrial abnormality; M-shaped P waves (P mitrale) are associated with left atrial abnormality.
- Ventricular chamber enlargement causes changes in the QRS complex.
- In right ventricular enlargement, the QRS complex in lead $V_1$ changes from negative to positive ($V_1$ begins to look like $V_6$); the QRS complex in lead $V_6$ changes from positive to negative ($V_6$ begins to look like $V_1$).
- In left ventricular enlargement, the voltage of the QRS complexes is exaggerated beyond normal (tall R waves grow taller and deep S waves grow deeper).
- Pulmonary embolus causes acute strain on the right heart and right axis deviation.
- Pericarditis represents a diffuse inflammatory process of the pericardial lining associated with widespread ST segment elevation. There is

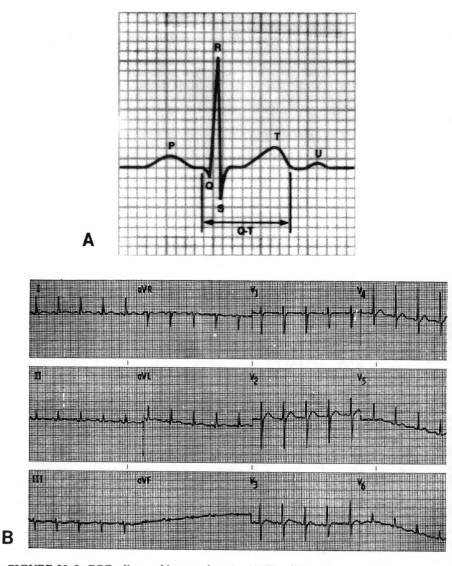

**FIGURE 20–9.** ECG effects of hypercalcemia. (*A*) The ST segment and QT intervals shorten with high levels of serum calcium. (From Dolan, JT: Critical Care Nursing: Clinical Management Through the Nursing Process. FA Davis, Philadelphia, 1991, p 826, with permission.) (*B*) The ST segment is virtually absent, resulting in a short QT interval in this example of hypercalcemia. (From Chung, EK: Electrocardiography: Practical Applications with Vectorial Principles, ed 3. Appleton & Lange, Norwalk, CT, 1985, p 532, with permission.)

usually an associated inflammation of the adjacent myocardium with pericarditis.

- Ventricular aneurysm causes persistent ST segment elevation.
- Ventricular aneurysm may be associated with mural thrombi and resistant ventricular dysrhythmias.
- Wolff-Parkinson-White (WPW) syndrome is a form of ventricular preexcitation that uses an accessory bypass tract.
- The classic ECG finding in WPW syndrome is a delta wave that slurs the initial QRS deflection.
- Chronic obstructive pulmonary disease (COPD) imposes chronic strain on the right heart and can result in ECG findings suggestive of right atrial abnormality and right ventricular enlargement.
- Cerebrovascular accident (CVA) causes repolarization changes on the ECG.
- Hypothermia causes myocardial depression.
- The Osborn wave is a classic ECG finding when core temperature is below 30°C.
- A positive exercise stress test causes either depression or (rarely) elevation of the ST segment and J point.
- False-positive results are commonly associated with exercise stress testing. Nuclear imaging increases the diagnostic sensitivity and specificity of the test.
- Stress testing with agents such as dipyridamole, adenosine, and dobutamine in conjunction with nuclear imaging or echocardiography are alternatives to conventional exercise testing in individuals who cannot exercise.
- The accuracy of Holter monitoring data is partly dependent on the accuracy of the patient diary.
- Orthotopic cardiac transplantation implies removal of the native heart and replacement with a donor heart.
- Remnant P waves are common after orthotopic cardiac transplantation.
- "Dig. effect" can cause predictable ECG changes such as prolongation of the PR interval and a "scooped out" ST segment.
- Digitalis toxicity causes dramatic ECG changes such as significant prolongation of the PR interval, varying degrees of AV block, and multiple dysrhythmias.
- Class I drugs can be proarrhythmic.
- Class IA drugs prolong the QT interval and widen the QRS complex.
- Class IB drugs shorten the QT interval.
- Class IC drugs prolong the PR, QRS, and QT intervals.
- Hypokalemia and hypomagnesemia cause prominent u waves.
- Hyperkalemia and hypermagnesemia cause tall, peaked T waves.
- Hypocalcemia lengthens the ST segment and QT interval.
- Hypercalcemia shortens the ST segment and QT interval.

# BIBLIOGRAPHY

American College of Cardiology/American Heart Association Task Force: Guidelines for implantation of cardiac pacemakers and antiarrhythmia devices: A report of the American College of Cardiology/American Heart Association task force on assessment of diagnostic and therapeutic cardiovascular procedures (committee on pacemaker implantation). J Am Coll Cardiol 18(1):1, 1991.

American Heart Association: Textbook of Advanced Cardiac Life Support, ed 2. American Heart Association, Dallas, 1990.

Arcebal, AG and Lemberg, L: Torsade de pointes. Heart Lung 9(6):1096, 1980.

Barbiere, CC and Liberatore, K: Automated external defibrillators: An update of additions to the ACLS algorithms. Crit Care Nurse June:17, 1992.

Brown, KR and Jacobson, S: Mastering dysrhythmias: A problem-solving guide. FA Davis, Philadelphia, 1988.

Callahan, ML: High-dose epinephrine therapy and other advances in treating cardiac arrest. West J Med 152:697, 1990.

Cascio, T: Nursing management of adults with common complications of cardiac disease. In Beare, PG and Myers, JL, (eds): Principles and Practice of Adult Health Nursing. CV Mosby, St. Louis, 1990.

Chernow, B (ed): Essentials of Critical Care Pharmacology. Baltimore, Williams & Wilkins, 1987.

Chung, EK: Electrocardiography: Practical Applications with Vectorial Principles, ed 3. Appleton & Lange, Norwalk, CT, 1985.

Conover, MB: Understanding Electrocardiography: Arrhythmias and the 12-Lead ECG, ed 5. CV Mosby, St. Louis, 1988.

DeBorde, R, Aarons, D, and Biggs, M: The automated implantable cardioverter. AACN Clin Issues in Crit Care Nurs 2(1):170, 1991.

Dunn, MI and Lipman, BS: Lipman-Massie Clinical Electrocardiography, ed 8. Year Book Medical Publishers, Chicago, 1989.

Emergency Cardiac Care Committee and Subcommittees, American Heart Association: Guidelines for cardiopulmonary resuscitation and emergency cardiac care. JAMA 268(16):2171, 1992.

Finkelmeier, NE: Pacemaker technology: An overview. AACN Clin Issues in Crit Care Nurs 2(1):99, 1991.

Halfman-Franey, M and Coburn, C: Techniques in cardiac care: lasers, stents, and atherectomy devices. AACN Clin Issues in Crit Care Nurs 1(1):87, 1990.

Lefor, N, Cardello, FP, and Felicetta, JV: Recognizing and treating torsade de pointes. Crit Care Nurse June:23, 1992.

Lipman, BC and Lipman, BS: ECG Pocket Guide. Year Book Medical Publishers, Chicago, 1987.

Lounsbury, P and Frye, SJ: Cardiac Rhythm Disorders: A Nursing Process Approach, ed 2. Mosby-Year Book, Inc., St. Louis, 1992.

Marriott, HJL: Practical Electrocardiography, ed 8. Williams & Wilkins, Baltimore, 1988.

Marriott, HJL and Conover, MB: Advanced Concepts in Arrhythmias, ed 2. CV Mosby, St Louis, 1989.

Morton, HS: Rate-responsive cardiac pacemakers. AACN Clin Issues in Crit Care Nurs 2(1):140, 1990.

Moser, DK, Woo, MA, and Stevenson, WG: Noninvasive identification of patients at risk for ventricular tachycardia with the signal-averaged electrocardiogram. AACN Clin Issues in Crit Care Nurs 1(1):79, 1990.

Opie, LH (ed): Drugs for the Heart, ed 3. WB Saunders, Philadelphia, 1991.

Physician's Desk Reference. Medical Economics Data, Montvale, NJ, 1992.

Roden, DM: Magnesium treatment of ventricular dysrhythmias. Am J Cardiol 63:43G, 1989.

Schactman, M and Greene, J: Signal-averaged electrocardiography: A new technique for determining which patients may be at risk for sudden death. Focus Crit Care 18(3):202, 1991.

Vallerand, AH and Deglin, JH: Drug Guide for Critical Care and Emergency Nursing. FA Davis, Philadelphia, 1991.

Vallerand, AH and Deglin, JH: Nurse's Guide for IV Medications. FA Davis, Philadelphia, 1991.

Vinsant, MO and Spence, MI: Commonsense Approach to Coronary Care: A Program, ed 5. CV Mosby, St Louis, 1989.

Waggoner, PC: Transcutaneous cardiac pacing. AACN Clin Issues in Crit Care Nurs 2(1):118, 1991.

Walraven, G: Basic Arrhythmias, ed 2 (rev). Brady Publishing, Englewood Cliffs, NJ, 1986.

Wilson, RF: Critical Care Manual: Applied Physiology and Principles of Therapy, ed 2. FA Davis, Philadelphia, 1992.

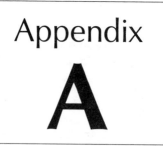

# Appendix

# A

# CARDIAC DRUGS
# ORAL AND INTRAVENOUS

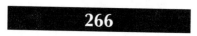

## ORAL CARDIAC DRUGS

| Drug | Indications | Mechanism | Dose | Special Points |
|------|-------------|-----------|------|----------------|
| Amiodarone (Cordarone) | Potentially life-threatening ventricular dysrhythmias unresponsive to conventional therapy | Class III antidysrhythmic agent; prolongs action potential; inhibits adrenergic stimulation | Supplied in 200-mg size Loading dose: 800–1600 mg/day × 1–3 weeks Maintenance dose: 600–800 mg qd × 4 weeks; then 400 mg qd | Half-life: 13–107 days; may be proarrhythmic; may cause pulmonary fibrosis, liver damage, and neuropathy; may increase serum levels of digoxin and class I drugs; monitor ECG for bradycardia and prolongation of PR, QRS, and QT |
| Atenolol (Tenormin) | Hypertension; angina pectoris; post MI treatment | Class II antidysrhythmic agent (cardioselective beta blocker); decreases HR and BP | Supplied in 50- and 100-mg sizes 25–150 mg qd | Monitor for development of bradycardia, hypotension, and/or CHF |
| Captopril (Capoten) | Hypertension; CHF; prevention of extension of infarct | ACE inhibitor (decreases BP) | Supplied in 12.5-, 25-, 50-, and 100-mg sizes 6.25–100 mg tid to qid | Do not give with food or antacids (decreases absorption); may cause orthostatic hypotension |
| Digoxin (Lanoxin, Lanoxicaps) | CHF; to slow ventricular rate in atrial fibrillation and atrial flutter; to terminate PSVT | Parasympathetic agonist (slows HR and conduction through the AV node); positive inotropic agent (enhances CO) | Lanoxin: Supplied in 0.125-, 0.25-, and 0.5-mg sizes Loading dose: 0.25–0.5 mg; then 0.25 mg q4 hr × 2 Maintenance: Variable | Avoid administration within 2 hr of antacid ingestion; may be proarrhythmic |

# ORAL CARDIAC DRUGS (Continued)

| Drug | Indications | Mechanism | Dose | Special Points |
|------|-------------|-----------|------|----------------|
| | | | Lanoxicaps: Supplied in 0.05, 0.1-, and 0.2-mg sizes<br>Loading dose: 0.4–0.6 mg; then 0.1–0.3 mg q6–8 hr × 2<br>Maintenance: Variable | Watch for bradycardia or CHF |
| **Diltiazem (Cardizem)** | Angina pectoris, coronary vasospasm; hypertension; non–Q wave MI; control of ventricular rate in SVT; hypertrophic cardiomyopathy | Class IV antidysrhythmic agent (calcium blocker); slows conduction through the AV node; vasodilates | Supplied in 30-, 60-, 90-, and 120-mg sizes<br>30–120 mg tid or qid | |
| **Disopyramide (Norpace, Norpace CR)** | Ventricular and supraventricular dysrhythmias | Class IA antidysrhythmic agent | Norpace: Supplied in 100- and 150-mg sizes<br>100–200 mg q6 hr<br>Norpace CR: Supplied in 100 and 150-mg sizes | Give on an empty stomach; monitor for CHF; may cause torsade de pointes; may cause dry mouth and urinary retention |
| **Enalapril (Vasotec)** | Hypertension; CHF; to reduce infarct size in acute MI | ACE inhibitor (decreases BP) | 200–400 mg q12 hr<br>Supplied in 2.5-, 5-, 10-, and 20-mg sizes<br>2.5–40 mg/day | Monitor for hypotension, especially after the first dose |
| **Encainide (Enkaid)** | Supraventricular dysrhythmias (special indication) and ventricular dysrhythmias (special indication) | Class IC antidysrhythmic agent (decreases automaticity, increases refractory period) | Supplied in 25-, 35-, and 50-mg sizes<br>25–50 mg q8 hr | May be proarrhythmic |

| Drug | Indications | Action | Dosage | Nursing Considerations |
|---|---|---|---|---|
| **Flecainide (Tambocor)** | Supraventricular dysrhythmias (special indication) and ventricular dysrhythmias (special indication) | Class IC antidysrhythmic agent (slows conduction, decreases automaticity, increases refractory period) | Supplied in 50-, 100-, and 150-mg sizes 50–100 mg q12 hr up to 400 mg qd | May be proarrhythmic |
| **Metoprolol (Lopressor)** | Angina pectoris; hypertension; supraventricular dysrhythmias; acute MI (after IV loading); hypertrophic cardiomyopathy | Class II antidysrhythmic agent (cardioselective beta blocker); decreases HR and CO | Supplied in 50- and 100-mg sizes 25–450 mg qd in divided doses | Give with food; monitor for bradycardia or CHF |
| **Mexiletine (Mexitil)** | Ventricular dysrhythmias | Class IB antidysrhythmic agent (decreases refractory period, decreases duration of the action potential) | Supplied in 150-, 200-, and 250-mg sizes 200–400 mg tid up to 1200 mg/day | Give with food; monitor for liver dysfunction |
| **Nadolol (Corgard)** | Angina pectoris; hypertension; supraventricular dysrhythmias | Class II antidysrhythmic agent (noncardioselective beta blocker) | Supplied in 20-, 40-, 80-, 120-, and 160-mg sizes 40–120 mg qd up to 240 mg | Monitor for bradycardia and CHF; drug level increases with renal failure |
| **Nifedipine (Procardia)** | Angina pectoris due to coronary vasospasm; hypertension | Class IV antidysrhythmic agent (calcium blocker); vasodilates | Supplied in 10- and 20-mg sizes 10–40 mg tid or qid up to 160 mg qd | Monitor for CHF; may cause peripheral edema |
| **Phenytoin (Dilantin)** | Ventricular dysrhythmias (especially digitalis-induced); anticonvulsant | Class IB antidysrhythmic agent (decreases automaticity, enhances conduction through the AV node) | Supplied in 30- and 100-mg sizes 100 mg bid or qid | Give with food; avoid administration within 2 hr of antacid ingestion; monitor for blood dyscrasias |

**ORAL CARDIAC DRUGS** *(Continued)*

| Drug | Indications | Mechanism | Dose | Special Points |
|---|---|---|---|---|
| **Procainamide (Pronestyl, Procan SR)** | Supraventricular and ventricular dysrhythmias | Class IA antidysrhythmic agent (decreases automaticity and excitability) | Pronestyl: Supplied in 250-, 375-, and 500-mg sizes 250–1000 mg q3–6 hr Procan SR: Supplied in 250-, 500-, 750-, and 1000-mg sizes 500–1000 mg q6 hr | Give on an empty stomach; may be associated with torsade de pointes and drug-induced lupus syndrome |
| **Propafenone (Rhythmol)** | Ventricular dysrhythmias | Class IC antidysrhythmic agent (prolongs conduction through the AV node, reduces automaticity and triggered activity); some beta blocker activity | Supplied in 150- and 300-mg sizes 150 mg tid up to 300 mg tid | May be proarrhythmic |
| **Propranolol (Inderal)** | Angina pectoris; hypertension; supraventricular dysrhythmias; acute MI; hypertrophic cardiomyopathy | Class II antidysrhythmic agent (noncardioselective beta blocker); decreases HR and BP, slows conduction through the AV node | Supplied in 10-, 20-, 40-, 60-, and 80-mg sizes 10–80 mg tid or qid up to 320 mg/day | Give with food; monitor for bradycardia and CHF |
| **Quinidine sulfate** | Supraventricular and ventricular dysrhythmias | Class IA antidysrhythmic agent (decreases automaticity and excitability) | Supplied in 200- and 300-mg sizes APC/VPC: 200–300 mg q6–8 hr; PSVT: 400–600 mg q2–3 hr until converted; then 200–300 mg q6–8 hr | Give on an empty stomach; monitor for GI distress; may be associated with torsade de pointes |

270

| Drug | Indications | Action | Supply/Dosage | Nursing Considerations |
|---|---|---|---|---|
| **Sotalol (Betapace)** | Ventricular dysrhythmias | Class II (beta blocker) and class III (lengthens action potential duration) antidysrhythmic properties | Supplied in 80-, 160-, and 240-mg sizes 80 mg bid up to 320 mg qd (rarely up to 640 mg qd) | Watch for proarrhythmia, follow Q-T interval, reduce dose with renal insufficiency (predominantly excreted in urine) |
| **Timolol (Blocadren)** | Angina pectoris; hypertension; supraventricular dysrhythmias; acute MI; hypertrophic cardiomyopathy | Class II antidysrhythmic agent (noncardioselective beta blocker); decreases HR and BP, slows conduction through the AV node | Supplied in 5-, 10-, and 20-mg sizes 10–20 mg bid to maximum of 60 mg qd | Monitor for bradycardia and CHF |
| **Tocainide (Tonocard)** | Ventricular dysrhythmias | Class IB antidysrhythmic agent (decreases automaticity) | Supplied in 400- and 600-mg sizes 400–600 mg q8 hr up to 2400 mg qd | Give with food |
| **Verapamil (Isoptin, Calan)** | Angina pectoris; hypertension; control of SVT; hypertrophic cardiomyopathy | Class IV antidysrhythmic agent (calcium blocker); slows HR; vasodilates | Supplied in 40-, 80-, and 120-mg sizes 40–120 mg tid or qid, up to 480 mg/day | Give with food; monitor for bradycardia and CHF |

HR = heart rate; BP = blood pressure; MI = myocardial infarction; CHF = congestive heart failure; AV = atrioventricular; SVT = supraventricular tachycardia; PSVT = paroxysmal supraventricular tachycardia; ACE = angiotensin-converting enzyme; CO = cardiac output; ECG = electrocardiogram; IV = intravenous; APC = atrial premature complex; VPC = ventricular premature complex; GI = gastrointestinal; qd = once a day; bid = two times a day; tid = three times a day; qid = four times a day.

**NOTE:** Information applicable to adult patients only. Unless otherwise indicated, dosages are for treatment of dysrhythmias only. Consult a pharmacology reference for an in-depth explanation of indications, contraindications, dosages, administration guidelines, side effects, and patient teaching concerns.

# INTRAVENOUS CARDIAC DRUGS

| Drug | Indication | Mechanism | Dose | Special Points |
|---|---|---|---|---|
| **Adenosine (Adenocard)** | Narrow QRS complex PSVT | Slows conduction through the AV node; interrupts reentry pathways in the AV node | 6 mg IVP over 1–3 sec (follow with 20 ml NS flush), if no response in 1–2 min, then 12 mg rapid IVP | Can be used to determine origin of wide-QRS tachycardia (ineffective in presence of VT); has short half-life (<5 sec); may produce transient bradycardia and ventricular ectopy |
| **Amrinone (Inocor)** | CHF | Positive inotropic agent (increases CO); vasodilator (decreases preload and afterload) | Loading dose: 0.75 mg/kg IV over 2–3 min, may repeat after 30 min. Maintain infusion at 5–15 µg/kg/min (titrate to response) | Avoid mixing in dextrose; incompatible with furosemide; may exacerbate myocardial ischemia or worsen ventricular ectopy |
| **Atropine** | Symptomatic bradydysrhythmias, asystole | Parasympathetic blocker (increases HR) | Do not exceed 10 mg/kg qd 0.5–1.0 mg IVP, repeat q3–5 min as needed (max dose = 3 mg) | If IV access delayed in arrest situation, may give via ET route (dilute in 10 ml NS or sterile water, use 2–2.5 × IV dose); use alternative agent to treat bradycardia in denervated heart; may increase myocardial oxygen demand; associated with urinary retention |
| **Bretylium (Bretylol)** | VF, VT, and other ventricular dysrhythmias resistant to conventional therapy | Class III antidysrhythmic agent; inhibits release of norepinephrine; vasodilator | VF: 5 mg/kg IVP (undiluted), if no response repeat 10 mg/kg IVP; maintain infusion at 1–2 mg/min (do not exceed 30–35 mg/kg/day) | Rapid IV administration may cause nausea and vomiting (if patient alert, give IVPB over 8–10 min); associated with hypotension; avoid in digoxin toxicity |

| Drug | Use | Action | Dose | Considerations |
|---|---|---|---|---|
| **Digoxin (Lanoxin)** | Controls ventricular rate in atrial flutter and atrial fibrillation; PSVT; CHF | Parasympathetic agonist (slows HR); slows conduction through the AV node; positive inotropic agent (enhances CO) | Loading dose: 0.25–0.5 mg slow IVP, then 0.25 mg IVP q2–4 hr | Can be proarrhythmic; correct hypovolemia and hypokalemia; serum levels increase with verapamil, quinidine, amiodarone |
| **Digoxin immune Fab (Digibind)** | Overdose of digitalis preparations (especially in presence of digitalis-induced dysrhythmias) | Antibody binds with free (unbound) digoxin so it cannot bind to cellular receptors | Unknown digoxin dose: 800 mg<br>Known digoxin dose: total body load × 66.7 = dose in mg (infuse through a filter over 30 min except in life-threatening situations; then give IVP) | Digoxin level increases after administration (represents digoxin bound to antibody fragments, so level may be misleading) |
| **Diltiazem (Cardizem)** | Controls ventricular rate in atrial flutter and atrial fibrillation; converts PSVT | Class IV antidysrhythmic agent (calcium blocker); slows conduction through the AV node; vasodilates | Loading dose: 0.25 mg/kg IVP over 2 min, after 15 min 0.35 mg/kg IVP over 2 min<br>Maintenance: 5–15 mg/hr | Watch for hypotension |
| **Dobutamine (Dobutrex)** | CHF | Adrenergic agonist (targets $\beta_1$ receptors, positive inotropic agent); at low doses increases CO without increasing HR | 2–20 $\mu$g/kg/min (titrate to response) | Correct hypovolemia; avoid extravasation |
| **Dopamine (Intropin)** | CHF; hypotension | Adrenergic agonist; effects are dose-specific: enhances renal flow at low doses; positive inotropic at moderate doses; vasoconstricts at high doses | 2–20 $\mu$g/kg/min (titrate to response, taper gradually) | Correct hypovolemia; inactivated in alkaline solutions; if >20 $\mu$g/kg/min required to maintain BP, consider giving with norepinephrine |

## INTRAVENOUS CARDIAC DRUGS (Continued)

| Drug | Indication | Mechanism | Dose | Special Points |
|------|-----------|-----------|------|----------------|
| **Epinephrine (Adrenalin)** | Ventricular fibrillation or asystole; hypotension; anaphylaxis | $\beta_1$ and $\beta_2$ agonist; positive inotropic and chronotropic effects; vasoconstricts; bronchodilates | VF/asystole: 1.0 mg (1:10,000 soln) IVP (if given peripherally follow with 20 ml NS flush), repeat q3–5 min as required<br>Maintenance: 1–4 µg/min (titrate to response) | If IV access delayed in arrest sitn, may give via ET route (dilute in 10 ml NS or sterile water, use 2–2.5 × IV dose); central route preferred; avoid mixing in alkaline solutions |
| **Esmolol (Brevibloc)** | Supraventricular tachycardia; hypertension associated with surgical procedures | Short-acting beta blocker (decreases HR, BP, contractility); slows conduction through the AV node | Loading dose: 500 µg/kg over 1 min followed by 50 mg/kg/min infusion over 4 min; may repeat sequence q5 min with an increase in maintenance infusion dose (do not exceed 200 µg/kg/min) | Monitor for hypotension; monitor for redness, swelling, burning at IV site |
| **Isoproterenol (Isuprel)** | Symptomatic bradydysrhythmias unresponsive to atropine; temporary control of hemodynamically significant bradycardia in denervated heart; refractory torsade de pointes | $\beta_1$ and $\beta_2$ agonist (increases HR and CO); vasodilates | Asystole and dysrhythmias: 2–10 µg/min (titrate to response) | May increase myocardial oxygen demand; avoid in acute mI |
| **Lidocaine (Xylocaine)** | Ventricular dysrhythmias | Class IB antidysrhythmic agent; decreases automaticity | Loading dose: 1–1.5 mg/kg IVP, may repeat 0.5–1.5 mg/kg IVP q5–10 min to a total of 3 mg/kg<br>Maintenance infusion at 1–4 mg/min (titrate) | If IV access delayed in arrest sitn, may give via ET route (dilute in 10 ml NS or sterile water); do not use to suppress ventricular escape beats; monitor for confusion, |

| Drug | Action | Indications | Dose | Nursing considerations |
|---|---|---|---|---|
| **Magnesium** | Electrolyte; plays a role in initiation and maintenance of cardiac muscle contraction | Hypomagnesemia (can precipitate dysrhythmias and pump failure); post-MI dysrhythmias; torsade de pointes | Refractory VT/VF: 1–2 g diluted in 100 ml D5W, infuse over 1–2 min<br>Post-MI: 1–2 g (8–16 mEq) in 50–100 ml D5W, infuse over 5–60 min, follow with 0.5–1.0 g/hr IV over 24 hr | visual disturbances, tremors; monitor drug levels; reduce dose after 24 hr<br>May cause hypotension or asystole |
| **Metoprolol (Lopressor)** | Class II antidysrhythmic agent (cardioselective beta blocker); decreases HR and CO | Supraventricular dysrhythmias; angina; hypertension; acute MI | Acute MI: 5 mg IVP q2 min × 3 doses; then 50 mg PO q 6 hr × 8 doses; then 100 mg PO bid | Monitor for bradycardia, hypotension, and CHF |
| **Nitroglycerin (Tridil)** | Vasodilator (venodilatation reduces preload); improves collateral flow to ischemic myocardium | Angina pectoris; acute MI; preload reduction in CHF; hypertension associated with surgical procedures | 5–20 $\mu$g/min and titrate upward to desired response | Prepare admixture in glass bottle, use nonpolyvinyl chloride tubing (drug may be absorbed into conventional polyvinyl chloride IV tubing); monitor for hypotension; correct hypovolemia |
| **Nitroprusside (Nipride)** | Vasodilator (arterial dilatation reduces afterload) | Hypertension (especially hypertensive crisis) afterload reduction in CHF | 0.5–10.0 $\mu$g/min (titrate to response) | Protect from light; monitor serum cyanate/thiocyanate levels; monitor for hypotension and metabolic acidosis; may exacerbate myocardial ischemia |
| **Norepinephrine (Levophed)** | $\alpha$ and $\beta_1$ agonist; vasoconstricts (increases BP); some positive inotropic effects (enhances CO) | Hypotension | 0.5–1.0 $\mu$g/min up to 30 $\mu$g/min (titrate to response) | Avoid extravasation (may cause tissue necrosis); do not infuse in alkaline solutions; correct hypovolemia |

## INTRAVENOUS CARDIAC DRUGS (Continued)

| Drug | Indication | Mechanism | Dose | Special Points |
|---|---|---|---|---|
| **Phenylephrine (Neo-Synephrine)** | Hypotension | α agonist (vasoconstricts); increases BP | Loading dose: 0.1–0.18 mg/min<br>Maintenance: 0.04–0.06 mg/min (titrate to response) | Avoid extravasation |
| **Phenytoin (Dilantin)** | Ventricular dysrhythmias, especially those that are digitalis induced; torsade de pointes | Class IB antidysrhythmic agent (decreases automaticity, enhances conduction through the AV node) | Loading dose: 50–100 mg q10–15 min up to 1 gr | Avoid administration in dextrose solutions (precipitate will form); rapid administration may cause hypotension and central nervous system depression |
| **Procainamide (Pronestyl)** | Atrial and ventricular dysrhythmias | Class IA antidysrhythmic agent (decreases automaticity and excitability) | Loading dose: 20 mg/min IVP up to 17 mg/kg<br>Maintenance: 1–4 mg/min | Monitor for hypotension and widening of the QRS complex during IV administration; may be associated with torsade de pointes |
| **Propranolol (Inderal)** | Angina pectoris; hypertension; supraventricular dysrhythmias; acute MI; hypertrophic cardiomyopathy | Class II antidysrhythmic agent (noncardioselective beta blocker); decreases HR and BP, slows conduction through the AV node | 0.5–3.0 mg IVP, may repeat in 2 min (then q4 hr) | Monitor for bradycardia and CHF |
| **Trimethaphan (Arfonad)** | Hypertension, especially acute crisis; aortic dissection | Sympathetic and autonomic ganglionic nerve blocker; vasodilates (decreases BP) | 0.5–6.0 mg/min, titrate slowly | May cause respiratory arrest |

| Verapamil (Isoptin, Calan) | Controls ventricular rate in atrial flutter and atrial fibrillation; terminates narrow QRS complex PSVT | Class IV antidysrhythmic agent (calcium blocker); slows conduction through the AV node | 2.5–5.0 mg IVP over 2 min, after 15–30 min may repeat 5–10 mg IVP over 2 min to a total of 20 mg | Monitor for hypotension and CHF; do not give in the presence of VT |

PSVT = paroxysmal supraventricular tachycardia; CHF = congestive heart failure; VF = ventricular fibrillation; VT = ventricular tachycardia; BP = blood pressure; HR = heart rate; IV = intravenous; IVP = intravenous push; IVPB = intravenous piggyback; AV = atrioventricular; CO = cardiac output; MI = myocardial infarction; NS = normal saline; ET = endotracheal tube.

**NOTE:** Information applicable to adult patients only. Unless otherwise indicated, dosages are for treatment of dysrhythmias only. Consult a pharmacology reference for an in-depth explanation of indications, contraindications, dosages, administration guidelines, side effects, and patient teaching concerns.

# Appendix

# B

## TABLE 1
## THE ALGORITHM APPROACH TO EMERGENCY CARDIAC CARE

These guidelines use algorithms as an educational tool. They are an illustrative method to summarize information. Providers of emergency care should view algorithms as a summary and a memory aid. They provide a way to treat a broad range of patients. Algorithms, by nature, oversimplify. The effective teacher and care provider will use them wisely, not blindly. Some patients may require care not specified in the algorithms. When clinically appropriate, flexibility is accepted and encouraged. Many interventions and actions are listed as "considerations" to help providers think. These lists should not be considered endorsements or requirements or "standard of care" in a legal sense. Algorithms do not replace clinical understanding. Although the algorithms provide a good "cookbook," the patient always requires a "thinking cook."

The following clinical recommendations apply to all treatment algorithms:

- First, treat the patient, not the monitor.
- Algorithms for cardiac arrest presume that the condition under discussion continually persists, that the patient remains in cardiac arrest, and that CPR is always performed.
- Apply different interventions whenever appropriate indications exist.
- The flow diagrams present mostly Class I (acceptable, definitely effective) recommendations. The footnotes present Class IIa (acceptable, probably effective), Class IIb (acceptable, possibly effective), and Class III (not indicated, may be harmful) recommendations.
- Adequate airway, ventilation, oxygenation, chest compressions, and defibrillation are more important than administration of medications and take precedence over initiating an intravenous line or injecting pharmacologic agents.
- Several medications (epinephrine, lidocaine, and atropine) can be administered via the endotracheal tube, but clinicians must use an endotracheal dose 2 to 2.5 times the intravenous dose.
- With a few exceptions, intravenous medications should always be administered rapidly, in bolus method.
- After each intravenous medication, give a 20- to 30-mL bolus of intravenous fluid and immediately elevate the extremity. This will enhance delivery of drugs to the central circulation, which may take 1 to 2 minutes.
- Last, treat the patient, not the monitor.

(Reproduced with permission, CPR Issue of *JAMA*, October 28, 1992. Copyright American Heart Association.)

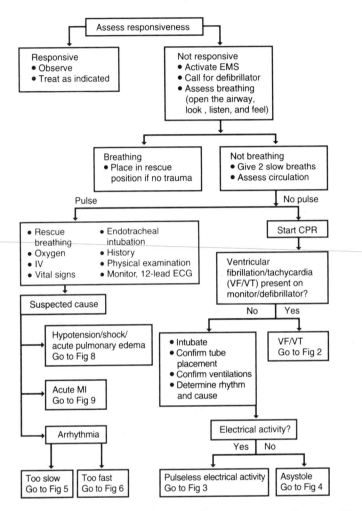

**FIGURE 1. The universal algorithm for adult emergency cardiac care.** The algorithm provides an overview of the rescuers' response in an emergency cardiac situation and integrates Basic Cardiac Life Support (BCLS) and Advanced Cardiac Life Support (ACLS). Emphasis is placed on rapid assessment of responsiveness, breathing, and circulation, with appropriate BCLS interventions. Once BCLS has been initiated, the rescuer is prompted to make clinical decisions regarding cardiac rhythms and hemodynamic status of the patient. Based on those decisions, the rescuer is directed to initiate the appropriate resuscitative approach as given in Figures 2 through 9 that follow. (Reproduced with permission, CPR Issue of *JAMA*, October 28, 1992. Copyright American Heart Association.)

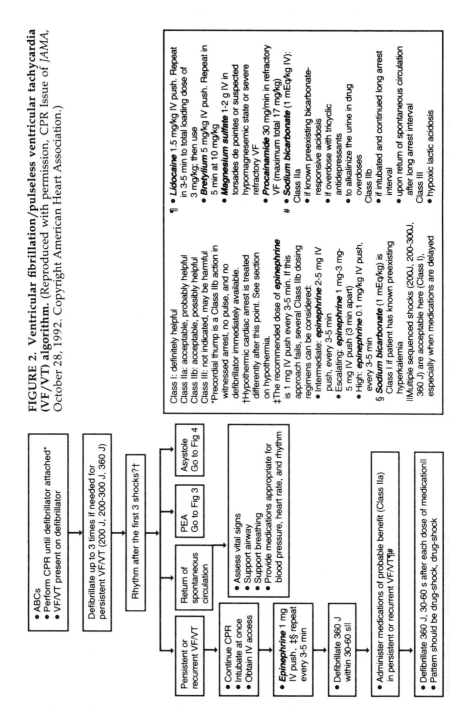

FIGURE 2. Ventricular fibrillation/pulseless ventricular tachycardia (VF/VT) algorithm. (Reproduced with permission, CPR Issue of *JAMA*, October 28, 1992. Copyright American Heart Association.)

- ABCs
- Perform CPR until defibrillator attached*
- VF/VT present on defibrillator

↓

Defibrillate up to 3 times if needed for persistent VF/VT (200 J, 200-300 J, 360 J)

↓

Rhythm after the first 3 shocks?†

→ Persistent or recurrent VF/VT
→ Return of spontaneous circulation
→ PEA — Go to Fig 3
→ Asystole — Go to Fig 4

Return of spontaneous circulation:
- Assess vital signs
- Support airway
- Support breathing
- Provide medications appropriate for blood pressure, heart rate, and rhythm

Persistent or recurrent VF/VT:
- Continue CPR
- Intubate at once
- Obtain IV access

↓

- *Epinephrine* 1 mg IV push, ‡§ repeat every 3-5 min

↓

- Defibrillate 360 J within 30-60 s‖

↓

- Administer medications of probable benefit (Class IIa) in persistent or recurrent VF/VT¶#

↓

- Defibrillate 360 J, 30-60 s after each dose of medication‖
- Pattern should be drug-shock, drug-shock

Class I: definitely helpful
Class IIa: acceptable, probably helpful
Class IIb: acceptable, possibly helpful
Class III: not indicated, may be harmful

*Precordial thump is a Class IIb action in witnessed arrest, no pulse, and no defibrillator immediately available.

†Hypothermic cardiac arrest is treated differently after this point. See section on hypothermia.

‡The recommended dose of *epinephrine* is 1 mg IV push every 3-5 min. If this approach fails, several Class IIb dosing regimens can be considered:
- Intermediate: *epinephrine* 2-5 mg IV push, every 3-5 min
- Escalating: *epinephrine* 1 mg-3 mg-5 mg IV push (3 min apart)
- High: *epinephrine* 0.1 mg/kg IV push, every 3-5 min

§ *Sodium bicarbonate* (1 mEq/kg) is Class I if patient has known preexisting hyperkalemia

‖Multiple sequenced shocks (200J, 200-300J, 360 J) are acceptable here (Class I), especially when medications are delayed

¶
- *Lidocaine* 1.5 mg/kg IV push. Repeat in 3-5 min to total loading dose of 3 mg/kg; then use
- *Bretylium* 5 mg/kg IV push. Repeat in 5 min at 10 mg/kg
- *Magnesium sulfate* 1-2 g IV in torsades de pointes or suspected hypomagnesemic state or severe refractory VF
- *Procainamide* 30 mg/min in refractory VF (maximum total 17 mg/kg)
- *Sodium bicarbonate* (1 mEq/kg IV):

Class IIa
- if known preexisting bicarbonate-responsive acidosis
- if overdose with tricyclic antidepressants
- to alkalinize the urine in drug overdoses

Class IIb
- if intubated and continued long arrest interval
- upon return of spontaneous circulation after long arrest interval

Class III
- hypoxic lactic acidosis

#

PEA includes
- Electromechanical dissociation (EMD)
- Pseudo-EMD
- Idioventricular rhythms
- Ventricular escape rhythms
- Bradyasystolic rhythms
- Postdefibrillation idioventricular rhythms

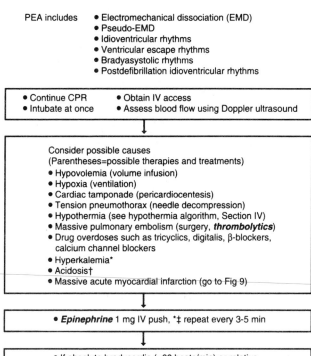

- Continue CPR
- Intubate at once
- Obtain IV access
- Assess blood flow using Doppler ultrasound

↓

Consider possible causes
(Parentheses=possible therapies and treatments)
- Hypovolemia (volume infusion)
- Hypoxia (ventilation)
- Cardiac tamponade (pericardiocentesis)
- Tension pneumothorax (needle decompression)
- Hypothermia (see hypothermia algorithm, Section IV)
- Massive pulmonary embolism (surgery, *thrombolytics*)
- Drug overdoses such as tricyclics, digitalis, β-blockers, calcium channel blockers
- Hyperkalemia*
- Acidosis†
- Massive acute myocardial infarction (go to Fig 9)

↓

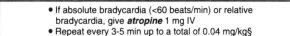

- *Epinephrine* 1 mg IV push, *‡ repeat every 3-5 min

↓

- If absolute bradycardia (<60 beats/min) or relative bradycardia, give *atropine* 1 mg IV
- Repeat every 3-5 min up to a total of 0.04 mg/kg§

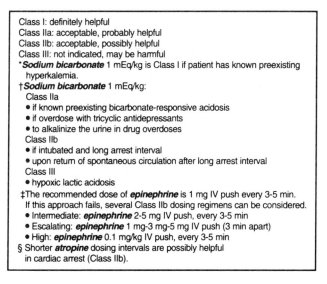

Class I: definitely helpful
Class IIa: acceptable, probably helpful
Class IIb: acceptable, possibly helpful
Class III: not indicated, may be harmful
*Sodium bicarbonate* 1 mEq/kg is Class I if patient has known preexisting hyperkalemia.
†*Sodium bicarbonate* 1 mEq/kg:
Class IIa
- if known preexisting bicarbonate-responsive acidosis
- if overdose with tricyclic antidepressants
- to alkalinize the urine in drug overdoses
Class IIb
- if intubated and long arrest interval
- upon return of spontaneous circulation after long arrest interval
Class III
- hypoxic lactic acidosis
‡The recommended dose of *epinephrine* is 1 mg IV push every 3-5 min. If this approach fails, several Class IIb dosing regimens can be considered.
- Intermediate: *epinephrine* 2-5 mg IV push, every 3-5 min
- Escalating: *epinephrine* 1 mg-3 mg-5 mg IV push (3 min apart)
- High: *epinephrine* 0.1 mg/kg IV push, every 3-5 min
§ Shorter *atropine* dosing intervals are possibly helpful in cardiac arrest (Class IIb).

**FIGURE 3. Pulseless electrical activity (PEA) algorithm.** (Reproduced with permission, CPR Issue of *JAMA*, October 28, 1992. Copyright American Heart Association.)

**FIGURE 4. Asystole treatment algorithm.** (Reproduced with permission, CPR Issue of *JAMA*, October 28, 1992. Copyright American Heart Association.)

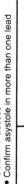
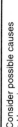

- Continue CPR
- Intubate at once
- Obtain IV access
- Confirm asystole in more than one lead

↓

Consider possible causes
- Hypoxia
- Hyperkalemia
- Hypokalemia
- Preexisting acidosis
- Drug overdose
- Hypothermia

↓

Consider immediate transcutaneous pacing (TCP)*

↓

- *Epinephrine* 1 mg IV push, †‡ repeat every 3-5 min

↓

- *Atropine* 1 mg IV, repeat every 3-5 min up to a total of 0.04 mg/kg§‖

↓

Consider
- Termination of efforts¶

Class I: definitely helpful
Class IIa: acceptable, probably helpful
Class IIb: acceptable, possibly helpful
Class III: not indicated, may be harmful

*TCP is a Class IIb intervention. Lack of success may be due to delays in pacing. To be effective TCP must be performed early, simultaneously with drugs. Evidence does not support routine use of TCP for asystole.

†The recommended dose of *epinephrine* is 1 mg IV push every 3-5 min. If this approach fails, several Class IIb dosing regimens can be considered:
- Intermediate: *epinephrine* 2-5 mg IV push, every 3-5 min
- Escalating: *epinephrine* 1 mg-3 mg-5 mg IV push (3 min apart)
- High: *epinephrine* 0.1 mg/kg IV push, every 3-5 min

‡*Sodium bicarbonate* 1 mEq/kg is Class I if patient has known preexisting hyperkalemia.

§Shorter *atropine* dosing intervals are Class IIb in asystolic arrest.

‖*Sodium bicarbonate* 1 mEq/kg:
Class IIa
- if known preexisting bicarbonate-responsive acidosis
- if overdose with tricyclic antidepressants
- to alkalinize the urine in drug overdoses
Class IIb
- if intubated and continued long arrest interval
- upon return of spontaneous circulation after long arrest interval
Class III
- hypoxic lactic acidosis

¶If patient remains in asystole or other agonal rhythms after successful intubation and initial medications and no reversible causes are identified, consider termination of resuscitative efforts by a physician. Consider interval since arrest.

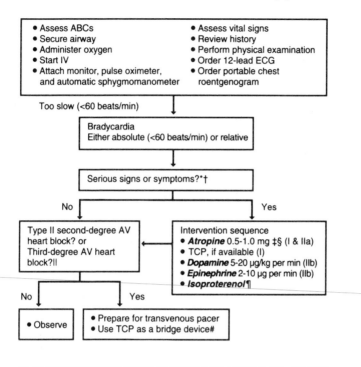

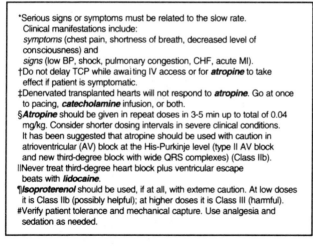

*Serious signs or symptoms must be related to the slow rate.
Clinical manifestations include:
*symptoms* (chest pain, shortness of breath, decreased level of consciousness) and
*signs* (low BP, shock, pulmonary congestion, CHF, acute MI).
†Do not delay TCP while awaiting IV access or for *atropine* to take effect if patient is symptomatic.
‡Denervated transplanted hearts will not respond to *atropine*. Go at once to pacing, *catecholamine* infusion, or both.
§*Atropine* should be given in repeat doses in 3-5 min up to total of 0.04 mg/kg. Consider shorter dosing intervals in severe clinical conditions. It has been suggested that atropine should be used with caution in atrioventricular (AV) block at the His-Purkinje level (type II AV block and new third-degree block with wide QRS complexes) (Class IIb).
‖Never treat third-degree heart block plus ventricular escape beats with *lidocaine*.
¶*Isoproterenol* should be used, if at all, with extreme caution. At low doses it is Class IIb (possibly helpful); at higher doses it is Class III (harmful).
#Verify patient tolerance and mechanical capture. Use analgesia and sedation as needed.

**FIGURE 5.  Bradycardia algorithm (patient not in cardiac arrest).** (Reproduced with permission, CPR Issue of *JAMA,* October 28, 1992. Copyright American Heart Association.)

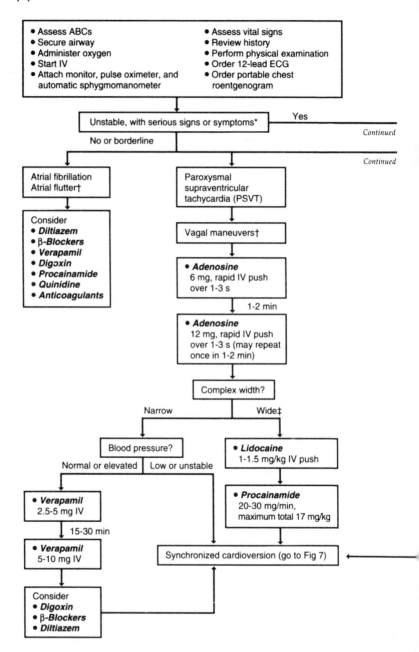

**FIGURE 6. Tachycardia algorithm.** (Reproduced with permission, CPR Issue of *JAMA*, October 28, 1992. Copyright American Heart Association.)

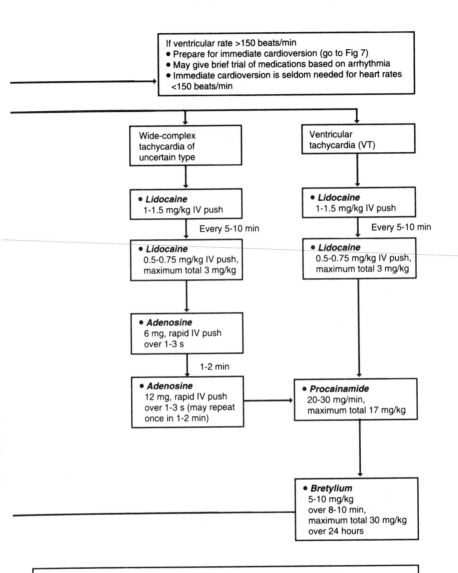

**If ventricular rate >150 beats/min**
- Prepare for immediate cardioversion (go to Fig 7)
- May give brief trial of medications based on arrhythmia
- Immediate cardioversion is seldom needed for heart rates <150 beats/min

| Wide-complex tachycardia of uncertain type | Ventricular tachycardia (VT) |

- *Lidocaine* 1-1.5 mg/kg IV push

Every 5-10 min

- *Lidocaine* 0.5-0.75 mg/kg IV push, maximum total 3 mg/kg

- *Lidocaine* 1-1.5 mg/kg IV push

Every 5-10 min

- *Lidocaine* 0.5-0.75 mg/kg IV push, maximum total 3 mg/kg

- *Adenosine* 6 mg, rapid IV push over 1-3 s

1-2 min

- *Adenosine* 12 mg, rapid IV push over 1-3 s (may repeat once in 1-2 min)

- *Procainamide* 20-30 mg/min, maximum total 17 mg/kg

- *Bretylium* 5-10 mg/kg over 8-10 min, maximum total 30 mg/kg over 24 hours

*Unstable condition must be related to the tachycardia. Signs and symptoms may include chest pain, shortness of breath, decreased level of consciousness, low blood pressure (BP), shock, pulmonary congestion, congestive heart failure, acute myocardial infarction.
†Carotid sinus pressure is contraindicated in patients with carotid bruits; avoid ice water immersion in patients with ischemic heart disease.
‡If the wide-complex tachycardia is known with certainty to be PSVT and BP is normal/elevated, sequence can include *verapamil*.

**FIGURE 6.** (*Continued.*)

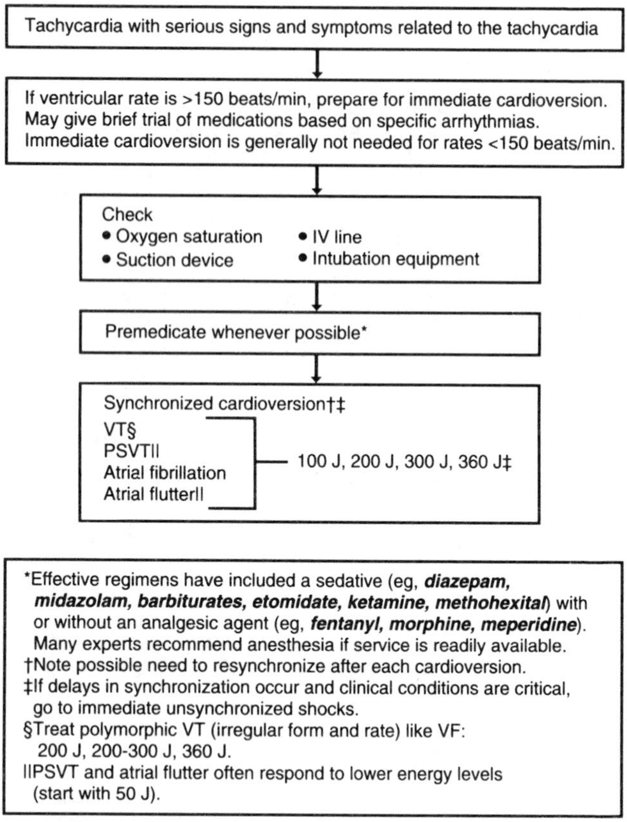

Tachycardia with serious signs and symptoms related to the tachycardia

↓

If ventricular rate is >150 beats/min, prepare for immediate cardioversion.
May give brief trial of medications based on specific arrhythmias.
Immediate cardioversion is generally not needed for rates <150 beats/min.

↓

Check
- Oxygen saturation    • IV line
- Suction device       • Intubation equipment

↓

Premedicate whenever possible*

↓

Synchronized cardioversion†‡
VT§
PSVT‖
Atrial fibrillation ⎱—— 100 J, 200 J, 300 J, 360 J‡
Atrial flutter‖

---

*Effective regimens have included a sedative (eg, **diazepam, midazolam, barbiturates, etomidate, ketamine, methohexital**) with or without an analgesic agent (eg, **fentanyl, morphine, meperidine**). Many experts recommend anesthesia if service is readily available.
†Note possible need to resynchronize after each cardioversion.
‡If delays in synchronization occur and clinical conditions are critical, go to immediate unsynchronized shocks.
§Treat polymorphic VT (irregular form and rate) like VF:
    200 J, 200-300 J, 360 J.
‖PSVT and atrial flutter often respond to lower energy levels (start with 50 J).

**FIGURE 7. Electrical cardioversion algorithm (patient not in cardiac arrest).**
(Reproduced with permission, CPR Issue of *JAMA*, October 28, 1992. Copyright American Heart Association.)

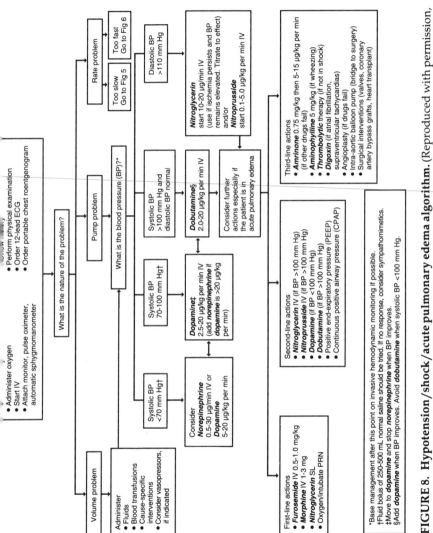

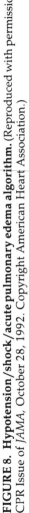

**FIGURE 8. Hypotension/shock/acute pulmonary edema algorithm.** (Reproduced with permission, CPR Issue of *JAMA*, October 28, 1992. Copyright American Heart Association.)

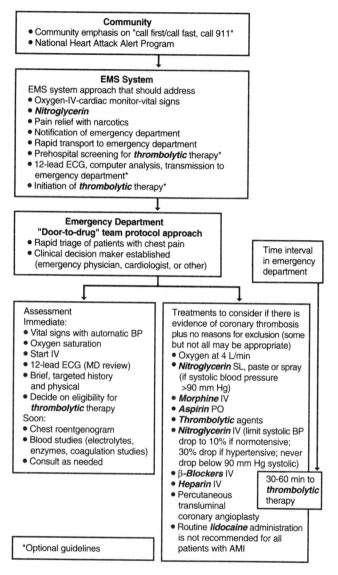

**Community**
- Community emphasis on "call first/call fast, call 911"
- National Heart Attack Alert Program

**EMS System**
EMS system approach that should address
- Oxygen-IV-cardiac monitor-vital signs
- *Nitroglycerin*
- Pain relief with narcotics
- Notification of emergency department
- Rapid transport to emergency department
- Prehospital screening for *thrombolytic* therapy*
- 12-lead ECG, computer analysis, transmission to emergency department*
- Initiation of *thrombolytic* therapy*

**Emergency Department**
**"Door-to-drug" team protocol approach**
- Rapid triage of patients with chest pain
- Clinical decision maker established (emergency physician, cardiologist, or other)

Time interval in emergency department

Assessment
Immediate:
- Vital signs with automatic BP
- Oxygen saturation
- Start IV
- 12-lead ECG (MD review)
- Brief, targeted history and physical
- Decide on eligibility for *thrombolytic* therapy
Soon:
- Chest roentgenogram
- Blood studies (electrolytes, enzymes, coagulation studies)
- Consult as needed

Treatments to consider if there is evidence of coronary thrombosis plus no reasons for exclusion (some but not all may be appropriate)
- Oxygen at 4 L/min
- *Nitroglycerin* SL, paste or spray (if systolic blood pressure >90 mm Hg)
- *Morphine* IV
- *Aspirin* PO
- *Thrombolytic* agents
- *Nitroglycerin* IV (limit systolic BP drop to 10% if normotensive; 30% drop if hypertensive; never drop below 90 mm Hg systolic)
- β-*Blockers* IV
- *Heparin* IV
- Percutaneous transluminal coronary angioplasty
- Routine *lidocaine* administration is not recommended for all patients with AMI

30-60 min to *thrombolytic* therapy

*Optional guidelines

FIGURE 9. Acute myocardial infarction (AMI) algorithm (recommendations for early treatment of patients with chest pain and possible AMI). (Reproduced with permission, CPR Issue of *JAMA*, October 28, 1992. Copyright American Heart Association.)

# Index

An f following a number indicates a figure on that page related to the topic given.

292Index

Isoproterenol, 274
Isoptin, 271, 277
Isuprel, 274
IVR. *See* Idioventricular rhythm

J wave, 238f, 239
James bypass tract, 236
JPC. *See* Junctional premature complex
J-point, 43, 48, 48f, 240–241
Junctional dysrhythmias, 114–119
Junctional escape rhythm, 58
Junctional premature complex (JPC), 114–116, 115f
Junctional rhythm, 58, 116–119, 116f, 118f, 211–212
  accelerated, 117–119, 118f
Junctional tachycardia, 117–119, 118f

Lanoxicap, 267
Lanoxin, 267, 273
Lateral limb leads, 74, 74f
Lateral wall myocardial infarction, 202, 203f
LBBB. *See* Left bundle branch block
Lead(s)
  I, 17, 17f, 77–80, 77f, 78f, 79f, 81f
  II, 17, 17f, 82f, 83f, 84f
  III, 17, 17f
  aVF, 14, 14f, 18, 18f, 73, 73f, 79–81, 79f, 81f
  aVL, 14, 14f, 18, 18f, 73, 73f, 82f, 83f, 84f
  aVR, 14, 14f, 18, 18f, 73, 73f
  axis, 71–72, 71f, 73, 73f
  bipolar limb, 17, 17f
  esophageal, 22, 22f
  group analysis, 201
  inferior limb, 74, 74f
  intra-atrial, 23
  lateral limb, 74, 74f
  Lewis, 22
  limb, 14, 14f, 17, 17f, 74, 74f
  localizing, 74, 74f
  MCL1-MCL6, 20, 20f
  modified chest (MCL), 20, 20f
  precordial, 14
  twelve-lead ECG, 14, 14f, 195, 200
  unconventional, 22–23, 22f
  unipolar limb, 18, 18f
  V1-V6, 14, 14f, 16, 16f, 19, 19f, 51–55, 51f, 53f, 55f, 204, 225
  *see also* Electrode(s)
Left anterior fascicular block (LAFB), 165–167, 166f, 169
Left atrial enlargement, 220, 222f, 223f, 261
Left axis deviation, 75f, 76, 85
Left bundle branch, 12, 12f
Left bundle branch block (LBBB), 162–164, 163f

Left posterior fascicular block (LPFB), 167–169, 167f
Left ventricular enlargement, 225–228, 226f, 227f, 261
Levophed, 275
Lewis lead, 22
Lidocaine, 274
Limb electrodes, 15, 15f
Limb leads, 14, 14f, 17, 17f, 74, 74f
Localizing leads, 74, 74f
Lopressor, 269, 275
Lown-Ganong-Levine syndrome, 236
LPFB. *See* Left posterior fascicular block

Macroreentry circuit, 104
Magnesium, 275
Mahaim bypass tract, 236
MAT. *See* Multifocal atrial tachycardia
MCL. *See* Modified chest leads
Mechanical contraction, 7, 7f, 25, 25f, 211
Metoprolol, 269, 275
Mexiletine, 269
Mexitil, 269
MI. *See* Myocardial infarction
Microreentry circuit, 103
Mobitz type I. *See* Atrioventricular (AV) blocks, second-degree type I
Mobitz type II. *See* Atrioventricular (AV) blocks, second-degree type II
Modified chest leads (MCL), 20, 20f
Multifocal atrial tachycardia (MAT), 102–103, 102f, 236
Multifocal ventricular premature complex. *See* Multiform ventricular premature complex
Multiform ventricular premature complex, 122, 124f
Mural thrombus, 233, 263
Muscle cell, 26, 26f
Myocardial depression, 263
Myocardial infarction (MI), 195–215
  acute, 207–208, 207f, 208f, 211–214
  anterior wall, 201, 202f
  ECG changes, 195–200, 196f, 207–208, 207f, 208f
  inferior wall, 204, 205f
  lateral wall, 202, 203f
  localization, 200–206
  non-Q-wave, 209–210, 209f
  posterior wall, 205, 206f
  subendocardial, 209, 209f
  transmural, 209f, 210
Myocardial injury, 196–198, 196f, 198f, 200
Myocardial ischemia, 195–196, 196f, 197f

Nadolol, 269
Negative electrode, 19
Negative QRS, 78